THE BIG
HEALTHY
SOUP
DIET

Other books by Linda Lazarides

The Waterfall Diet
Treat Yourself with Nutritional Therapy
Amino Acid Report
Nutritional Health Bible
Principles of Nutritional Therapy
HIV Self-Help Manual

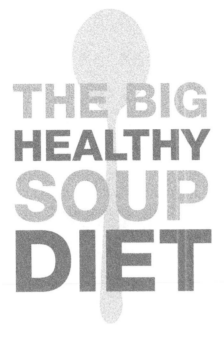

THE BIG HEALTHY SOUP DIET

Nourish Your Body and
Lose up to 10 lbs a Week

LINDA LAZARIDES

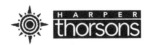

HARPER
thorsons

HarperThorsons
A Imprint of HarperCollins*Publishers*
77–85 Fulham Palace Road
Hammersmith, London W6 8JB

The website address is
www.thorsonselement.com

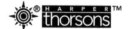

and *HarperThorsons* are trademarks of
HarperCollins*Publishers* Ltd

Published by HarperThorsons 2005

A catalogue record for this book is
available from the British Library

ISBN-13 978-0-00-720756-5

Find out more about HarperCollins and the environment at
www.harpercollins.co.uk/green

CONTENTS

INTRODUCTION:

HEALTH IN A BOWL – LOOK
AND FEEL GOOD WITH SOUP!

Whether you're trying to lose weight or just to get more healthy, soup is the ultimate convenience food: easy to make, filling and low in calories. Soup is never boring. It can be thick or thin, smooth or chunky, or a combination of the two. Healthy ingredients and power foods can be combined easily and deliciously to maximize weight-loss or combat ailments. If you want to lose weight, soup can help to release hidden water retention, control appetite, stimulate metabolism and promote fat-loss. You can add ingredients to promote the good health of arteries, bones, skin and hormones; or others to reduce blood pressure and cholesterol and fight the causes of arthritis. What more could you ask for from a meal? Is there no limit to what soup can do?

So how does it work? The Big Healthy Soup Diet is the ultimate food-combining system. It's all about putting in the right ingredients and power foods for what you want to achieve, and then waiting for the results. If you want to lose weight there's no need to choose between low-carb, low-calorie, detox, food-combining, glycaemic index, water-release or cabbage soup diets when you can have them all rolled into one. As a nutritionist, I find that soup gets you to your target weight faster and more easily than anything else. The ancient food-combining wisdom of Oriental and Ayurvedic medicine can also be applied to soup – it is so incredibly versatile. The recipes are all here for you. With the

Big Healthy Soup Diet you will learn how to lose not just excess body fat, but also hidden water retention, a common cause of excess weight that cannot be shifted with normal diets. The result is maximum weight-loss for minimum effort!

Many of the soups in this book make satisfying one-pot meals. Best of all, you can return for second helpings as you won't be piling on the calories. The warmth and liquid of soup fill you up quickly, and the recipes make extensive use of ingredients rich in soluble fibre. This means you get minimal calories while slowing down carbohydrate absorption, helping to prevent surges in the hormones that stimulate appetite.

If you are currently following a diet and don't feel ready just yet to make a change, don't worry – the Big Healthy Soup Diet has lots of recipes suitable for conventional low-carb and detox diets.

On the other hand, if you've bought this book just to be healthy, and don't need to lose weight, then simply add the soup recipes to your normal diet. A large bowl of soup can provide the recommended three servings a day of fresh vegetables, which help to prevent cancer and heart disease. And there are fruit soup recipes too. The recipes are full of power foods to help rejuvenate your body systems, balance your hormones and combat the effects of stress.

HOW TO USE THIS BOOK

The Big Healthy Soup Diet can help you to

- Reach your ideal weight and keep it there
- Prevent future illness
- Combat ailments or health problems
- Enjoy eating healthy foods

Losing Weight and Looking Good

Read Part I to find out how soup and its power ingredients can help you to lose weight. This section also gives two special health programmes. Programme 1 is a four-day mini-detox to help you clean out your system, shed some water retention and start getting into a more healthy state. Programme 2 is the 10-day Big Healthy Soup Diet to help you reach your ideal weight. Designed to help you shed both fat and water retention (a common cause of excess weight), this 10-day diet could enable you to lose up to 10 lbs.

Staying Healthy with Soup

Read Part II to find out about soups that can help you and your loved ones reach a ripe old age without too many visits to the doctor. We all know that you are what you eat, and how important it is to consume lots of vegetables. That's not always as easy as it sounds. But eating lots of delicious soups with the right ingredients makes it *so* much easier to cut down on foods with the wrong ones! This part of the book tells you about soups that can help to prevent high blood pressure, gallstones, memory loss and even breast cancer. It also reveals the latest amazing discoveries from the world's top research establishments.

Feeling Good with Soup

Part III is about using food as medicine. Thousands of doctors all over the world now specialize in this very effective way to treat problems with hormones, energy, bones, joints, nervous system and blood pressure. Eating the right soups could make all the difference. Soup can actually help to rejuvenate your glands, organs and other systems. It provides the intense nourishment needed in order to combat ailments more effectively. And what could be a more mouth-watering way to take your medicine?

Enjoy Eating Healthy Foods

Part IV of the Big Healthy Soup Diet is the delicious recipes. Turn straight to this section if you are just looking for a tasty starter or a one-pot meal. You are sure to find something tempting, and all the soups are bursting with goodness. Some are so quick and easy to make that you may never again buy soup in a can!

PART I

LOSING WEIGHT AND
LOOKING GOOD

WHY SOUP?

Although some weight-loss plans involve special techniques like cutting out carbohydrates, most people still tend to think of eating fruit and salads as the best way to lose weight. Apples, lettuce, cucumber and tomatoes are very low-calorie foods. You can fill up a whole plate with these items and still consume only 100 Calories. It seems logical that if you eat only 100 Calories for lunch, you must lose weight ... right?

Well, maybe. The big problem is that most people who use this approach can't stick with it for very long. After bingeing on chocolate a couple of times and giving up the diet in despair, these individuals (and you are probably one of them!) usually blame themselves for their 'weak willpower'.

In fact, we now know that there is a very good reason why this type of diet is doomed from the start. Salad foods are cold. Too much cold food can make you feel depressed, especially if you are a chilly individual and feel the cold easily. Depression is also a 'rebound' effect of excessive deprivation. It leads to an overwhelming desire for comfort

(1,000 calories = 1 Calorie or kilocalorie. Throughout this book the word 'calorie' refers to 'kilocalories'.)

foods – most of which are, of course, loaded with excess calories. This is a physical desire. It has nothing to do with being greedy or weak-willed. Your body is desperate to get warmth and energy and it forces you to crave foods that will quickly satisfy those needs. Modern weight-loss science is just beginning to recognize this problem, and to work with it rather than against it.

Traditional Oriental wisdom has understood the problem all along. In Oriental medicine, too much raw or cold food would be considered to encourage weight *gain* as it depletes the body's 'fire' or Yang energy (metabolism). Hot chunky soups made with lentils and moderately flavoured with garlic, onion, cayenne, chilli and ginger are much more energizing. Oriental experts believe that such foods burn off excess water in our bodies, and this is of course very good news for sufferers of water retention – a common cause of overweight. Don't overdo these spices – burning your insides would be counterproductive and unnecessary.

The warmth of soup makes you feel full as salad rarely can. Soup itself is a comfort food. But owing to its water content and healthy ingredients, this is a low-calorie comfort food and there is no problem with extra helpings. You won't eat any more calories than in the average salad. But the results are far superior:

- **Fewer cravings for sweet, starchy and fatty food**
- **Much improved ability to stick to the diet**
- **Faster, more successful weight-loss**

SOUP RESEARCH

Even scientific researchers agree that soup has some very special properties. In 1999, Barbara J. Rolls and Elizabeth A. Bell of Pennsylvania State University discovered that feeling full doesn't need to depend on the number of calories you eat. If you know how, you can feel full just by making each calorie more filling. How do you do this? By adding hot water to your food to make soup! In this study, 24 young women were fed a 270-calorie appetizer of chicken-rice casserole – first on its own, second with a glass of water, and finally by adding the glass of water to the casserole and serving it up as chicken-rice soup. Then the researchers measured how much lunch the women ate afterwards. The results were incredible. After the casserole or the casserole/glass of water they proceeded to consume 300 calories for lunch. But after a bowl of soup, they could only manage to eat 200 calories. That's a one-third reduction! *Nor did they get hungry earlier or eat a bigger dinner later!* It seems that when water is incorporated into food the body becomes satisfied much more easily.

This is a whole new area of weight-loss research, and several more studies are summarized at the end of this chapter. It is another interesting fact that, according to the research, chunky soups are more effective in controlling appetite than smooth, puréed soups. All this helps to explain the success of the Cabbage Soup Diet made famous by Dolly Parton. But cabbage also has some special properties of its own, as you will find out later. The Big Healthy Soup Diet includes five new and delicious recipes for cabbage soup.

INGREDIENTS THAT KEEP YOU FEELING FULL

With the right ingredients, soup can be even more satisfying and keep you full for even longer. It can also help to balance your hormones, and this is essential when you want to burn off your body fat.

Three ingredients that help weight-loss when added to soup include:

- Fats and oils
- Protein
- Soluble fibre

Fats and Oils

It's just so easy to say 'Fats and oils are high in calories so cut them out and you'll lose weight.' This only makes people start cutting out the fats they can *see*: butter and margarine, cream, cooking and salad oils, meat fat and even the skin from chickens. In fact, eaten in moderation, none of these are a problem. It is hidden fats – the fats you *can't* see –

that really pile on the pounds. Foods with large amounts of hidden fat include:

- Biscuits and cookies
- Burgers
- Cakes
- Chocolate
- Creamy dips
- Creamy desserts
- Crispy snacks
- Deep-fried food
- Ice cream
- Pies and pastries
- Sausages and salami

For instance, have you ever read a recipe for making chocolate brownies? Most brownie recipes contain even more fat and sugar than they do flour. Every portion of pastry or pie-crust you consume probably contains at least two tablespoons of pure fat. You can't see it, but just try pressing a few crumbs on a piece of paper and see the grease spots appear. Burgers can easily consist of up to 70 per cent invisible fat. Burger meat can quite legally be described as 'lean' even if it contains up to 30 per cent fat. Imagine how hard it is to lose weight if you keep eating too many foods like this. And imagine what they do to your skin – making it greasy and prone to blackheads as a result of clogged pores. Too much saturated fat also affects your blood circulation, and this is bad news for cells that make collagen. As you know, skin sags and shrinks when your collagen starts to deteriorate. You need to feed your collagen-making cells with the right food in order to stay looking young as long as possible.

High-fat foods also tend to make you feel sluggish. Vitality is attractive, but its opposite – sluggishness – is not!

The Big Healthy Soup Diet aims to make it easier for you to stop eating high-fat junk foods. One of its techniques is to include a healthy proportion of good quality oils, and occasionally even a little cream. When strictly controlled, these fats make weight-loss much easier.

They make your soups substantial, filling and delicious. If you find your-self craving junk food, have another helping of soup and the craving will be much less. It will cease to be a physical craving.

The hormone that makes you fat

Beware of trying to cut corners by cutting the oils out of the recipes in this book. It is tempting to think you might lose weight faster if you do, but there are several special reasons why you actually *need* these ingredients.

Fats or oils slow down your digestion and absorption of other food ingredients. This is why they help to control your appetite – food takes longer to get through your system when it contains a lit-tle fat or oil. Most importantly, fats or oils slow down your absorp-tion of starches and sugars (carbohydrates). This makes you produce insulin more slowly. Insulin is a hormone that carries out many tasks in the body. It is essential to help you turn carbohy-drates into energy, but you don't want to have too much of it hang-ing around. High insulin levels occur when you eat too much carbohydrate. They

- Raise your cholesterol levels
- Slow down your loss of body fat
- Encourage your body to turn calories into fat
- Encourage water retention (by slowing down your excretion of sodium)

Can you see why it is positively beneficial to have some fat or oil in your diet? But if your thoughts are now wandering towards a bar of chocolate, try to stop them. It is your meals (soup) that must contain the oil. Your meals must be as satisfying as possible so that you won't crave sugar and high-calorie snacks between meals. The fats or oils must also be nutritionally useful, providing monounsaturated or essential polyunsaturated oils, and the retinol (true vitamin A) and vitamin D that your body cannot get elsewhere. The meal must also be free of sugary items, since these will push up your insulin levels regardless of how much fat or oil you eat.

I hope it is becoming clear that there is a lot more to fats and oils than just calories. In fact, used in moderation as suggested in this book, oils should really be applauded because of their ability to control appetite and prevent excessive insulin surges. In moderation, some oils (such as olive oil) are also very healthy in their own right.

HEALTH BENEFITS OF OILS

Butter, cheese and cream provide retinol and vitamin D, needed by your bones, mucous membranes and immune system. It is difficult to get these nutrients elsewhere. Olive oil is known to have many health benefits and, like coconut oil, will combat harmful fungi which many people harbour in their intestines. Extra-virgin olive oil also contains an abundance of useful antioxidants. Soy and nut oils provide polyunsaturated fatty acids, which are vital for health. If you cut them out of your diet you can develop problems with your skin, hormones and water balance.

Protein

Protein as a weight-loss tool has been made famous by the Atkins diet. This diet cuts out carbohydrates and replaces them with protein, fats, oils and non-starchy fruit and vegetables. For a long time no-one really knew how the diet worked. Now that more research has been done, it is clear that people become full quite quickly when they eat mostly protein and fat, and they end up consuming smaller quantities of food and therefore fewer calories. By cutting out carbohydrates they also produce much lower levels of insulin and so avoid a major hormonal cause of weight-gain.

Protein is, of course, found in meat, fish and eggs. It is also a major ingredient of dairy and soy products, nuts, seeds, beans, chickpeas and lentils. Like fats and oils, protein takes quite a while to digest, so it keeps you feeling full for longer. But like carbohydrates, protein can also overstimulate insulin production if not consumed together with a little fat or oil.

Low-carb diets such as Atkins have gained a reputation that you *have* to eat a lot of protein. People are worried about this because too much protein dehydrates the body and makes it acidic. This acidity is harmful and stressful for your kidneys. In fact, low-carb diets don't have to contain harmfully high amounts of protein. Instead of eating sugar

---

BUTTER, CHEESE AND CREAM? BAD IN EXCESS BUT GOOD IN MODERATION!

Retinol is the true form of vitamin A, and is found only in dairy products, eggs, liver and oils extracted from the liver of fish such as cod and halibut. Forms of retinol are also artificially added to margarine.

Fruits and vegetables are said to contain vitamin A but really they don't. They do provide beta-carotene, which ideally should be converted to vitamin A in your upper intestines by the action of bile salts and fat-splitting enzymes. In fact, you have to eat quite a large amount of fruits and vegetables to make even your minimum vitamin A requirements, even assuming that all conditions in your body are ideal for the conversion.

Conditions are often not ideal. People with diabetes or an under-functioning thyroid (a common condition, often not diagnosed until much too late) cannot make any vitamin A from beta-carotene. Children also make the conversion very poorly and babies not at all, which is one reason why they must not be given low-fat milk. Excessive consumption of alcohol, iron pills, recreational drugs and polyunsaturated fats can interfere with the conversion. Zinc deficiency is common and is also detrimental.

Carotenes are converted to vitamin A by the action of bile salts, but very little bile is released when a meal is too low in fat or oil. On the other hand, butter and cream not only provide ready-made vitamin A but also stimulate the secretion of bile. Polyunsaturated oils also stimulate the secretion of bile salts but they can destroy carotene unless sufficient antioxidant vitamins are present.

and other carbohydrates, you can fill up on liquid and on masses of fruit and vegetables. This will both prevent dehydration and help to control your acidity levels. Soup provides both liquid and vegetables, so you can gain all the benefits of a low-carb diet while minimizing the side-effects.

In this book you will be consuming mostly healthy forms of protein: fish, organic poultry and dairy products, lentils, beans and tofu. Nuts and seeds such as sunflower and sesame seeds are also included – for both their protein and the beneficial oils they provide. Very few of the soup recipes contain red meat. This is because the fat associated with red meat is not healthy. Also, the World Health Organization has found that people who consume red meat more than twice a week have a higher risk of developing cancer.

It is much better to eat white meat and to supplement this with olive oil, nut oils and with retinol- and vitamin D-rich fats from milk, cheese and cream.

Soluble Fibre

Dietary fibre absorbs liquid and so helps to bulk up the contents of your intestinal tract. This keeps you feeling full for longer after a meal. Adding bran to your food was one of the features of the F-Plan diet, which became popular in the 1970s. 'F' stood for fibre, and the diet involved consuming as much fibre as possible because this would reduce the calorie content of your meal while still keeping you satisfied.

But bran is not an ideal fibre for this purpose. It contains a lot of phytic acid, which forms complexes with minerals in your food and prevents their absorption. In large amounts, bran can also be quite irritating to the intestines, and is prone to causing gas. Nowadays we are more likely to recommend soluble fibre as a dieting aid. Soluble fibre is found in seeds, lentils, beans, seaweed extracts, fruit and vegetables. Like bran, it is indigestible, but unlike bran, it can be consumed by bacteria in your intestines and turned into useful fatty acids, which maintain an ideal acidity balance in your colon and support the health of your colon walls.

One of the best forms of soluble fibre is pectin. Found mostly in apples, cabbage and the white part of citrus fruit, pectin holds up to

100 times its weight in water. This excellent bulking action is very helpful for controlling appetite, especially if the pectin is in warm foods such as cooked fruit soups and cabbage soup.

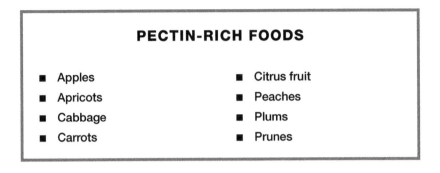

PECTIN-RICH FOODS

- Apples
- Apricots
- Cabbage
- Carrots

- Citrus fruit
- Peaches
- Plums
- Prunes

Several research studies have also shown that consuming a lot of pectin can lower your cholesterol levels. Pectin binds to bile acids (released by your liver into your intestines when fats and oils are consumed) and prevents you from reabsorbing them and turning them into cholesterol. Pectin also helps to keep bile flowing, and this is beneficial as it means your gall bladder (which stores bile) is regularly flushed out.

The success of the Cabbage Soup Diet may be partly due to the pectin content of cabbage. In this book you will find several soup recipes containing cabbage. These recipes help to make cabbage more interesting, and some of them use spices which enhance the weight-loss potential of this vegetable.

Psyllium husks (see Resources, page 277) can also be added to soup, and are a good thickener for soups such as *Chinese Hot and Sour Soup* (see page 224). These seed husks are an ancient Ayurvedic treatment for cleansing the intestines, and are extremely rich in a type of soluble fibre known as mucilage. Mucilage is also found in seaweed, and many commercial vegetarian gelling products such as agar-agar consist of mucilage extracted from seaweed. (Adding mucilage to liquids thickens and gels them.) Psyllium husks can do a similar job and are cheap and easy to use. Owing to their huge capacity for absorbing water in the intestines, and so helping to bulk out the stools, psyllium husks are used as the basis of many anti-constipation remedies. One tablespoon a day whisked into a large glass of water encourages regular bowel motions without causing discomfort or diarrhoea. Combined with soup, psyllium husks will absorb and gel much of the liquid, so to your stomach they will feel more like solid food and will help you to stay full for longer.

OTHER POWER FOODS TO AID WEIGHT-LOSS

In Ayurvedic and Oriental medicine, overweight is said to be caused by an excess of 'dampness' in the body. The dampness (fluid) quenches the body's fire (metabolism) and so encourages the laying down of fat. The Oriental treatment for obesity consists of drying out the dampness, using special foods that 'soak it up' or alternatively drive it out by boosting Yang energy to heat up the metabolism (see panel below).

YIN AND YANG

These are important concepts in Oriental medicine. Yang represents male qualities (such as hard, dry, dense, hot, pungent) and Yin represents feminine qualities (such as soft, damp, loose, cool, sweet). For good health these should always be in balance. If they become out of balance, eating the right foods can help to correct any associated problems.

Excessive dampness leading to overweight suggests that there is too much Yin energy in the body and not enough Yang, so eating aduki beans (which are hard, dense and dry before cooking) or pepper and garlic (which are respectively hot and pungent) helps to correct the imbalance.

Always bear in mind that Oriental medicine is about balance. So don't overdo the pepper and burn your insides thinking that this will help you lose weight faster. It won't!

Aduki beans and broad beans are considered good for soaking up dampness. The best part of the broad bean is the pod, and soup can be made with water in which the pods have been boiled. Mung beans and bean sprouts are also recommended if your weight problem is accompanied by an excessively hot constitution – that is to say if you feel the heat easily and suffer from skin eruptions.

To increase the Yang energy on which metabolism depends, Oriental medicine recommends the regular consumption of kidneys, liver (preferably from organically-raised livestock), shrimps and mussels.

Oriental medicine includes a great deal about increasing 'fire' or 'heat' in the body. Ayurvedic medicine also emphasizes the importance of supporting the 'digestive fire' in order to improve digestion and reduce unhealthy sedimentary deposits in the body's tissues. Is there a Western equivalent? Indeed there is. Many so-called warming herbs and spices create the sensation of warmth in the body (ginger and pepper in particular). They are well-known circulatory stimulants and can

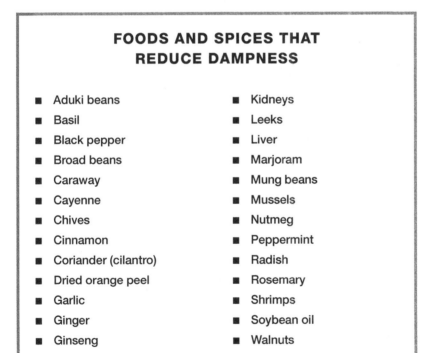

FOODS AND SPICES THAT
REDUCE DAMPNESS

- Aduki beans
- Basil
- Black pepper
- Broad beans
- Caraway
- Cayenne
- Chives
- Cinnamon
- Coriander (cilantro)
- Dried orange peel
- Garlic
- Ginger
- Ginseng

- Kidneys
- Leeks
- Liver
- Marjoram
- Mung beans
- Mussels
- Nutmeg
- Peppermint
- Radish
- Rosemary
- Shrimps
- Soybean oil
- Walnuts

induce sweating. When consumed, they warm the circulation in the digestive system and bring the blood to the surface of the intestinal wall where it can more easily absorb nutrients from the intestinal contents. This is highly beneficial for both good health and appetite control.

WATER RETENTION – AN IMPORTANT CAUSE OF OVERWEIGHT

The Oriental concept that overweight is caused by excessive damp-ness in the body is very interesting from a Western point of view. Not all excess body weight is fat. As pointed out in my book *The Waterfall Diet*, hidden water retention is extremely common and can add many pounds to the scales. From a Western viewpoint there are several causes of water retention, ranging from food intolerances (sometimes known as food 'allergies') to excessive salt consumption.

CAUSES OF UNEXPLAINED WATER RETENTION

- Food intolerances (allergies)
- Protein deficiency (usually in people on very low-calorie diets)
- Deficiencies of vitamin B6 and/or magnesium
- Lack of fruit and vegetables
- Lack of exercise
- Excessive salt consumption
- Anaemia
- Some medications
- Inflammation due to high toxin levels

Unexplained water retention can account for 10 lbs or more of excess body weight. If you eat the right foods all this water can be urinated away within a week!

The Waterfall Diet provides foods that help address these causes, and omits foods that could potentially contribute to water retention. Many of the soup recipes in this book are suitable for the Waterfall Diet (see the Index on page 131). If you want to see whether you need the Waterfall Diet, try consuming just these soups and nothing else for 10 days. If you spend a lot of time urinating and your clothes quickly begin to hang loose, then you definitely need to read more about the Waterfall Diet (see Resources, page 277) so that you can combat this problem on a more long-term basis.

If you have two or more of the following signs you may be suffering from water retention:

- You have worked hard to lose weight using conventional methods, and found that you cannot get below a certain weight even by persevering for months or years
- Pressing a fingernail firmly into your thumb-pad leaves a deep dent that won't go away after a second or two
- Pressing the tip of your finger into the inside of your shin-bone leaves a dent
- Swelling of legs, feet or ankles
- Your shoe size seems to increase as you get older
- Rings sometimes seem not to fit any more
- You seem to have a major swelling problem in hot weather
- Your tummy is often tight and swollen
- Breast tenderness (in women)
- Premenstrual weight gain (in women)
- Your weight fluctuates by several pounds within the space of only 24 hours

FOOD ADDICTIONS

If you have a lot of weight to lose, the good news is that the Big Healthy Soup Diet is ideal to help you. But of course there is more to weight-loss than just eating the right diet. Exercise (see page 17) is equally important. And, due to the well-known problem of food

ADVICE TO COMBAT FOOD ADDICTIONS

Don't miss meals. Missed meals lead to much greater cravings for addictive foods. Eat extra portions of soup for the first two weeks while you are going through sugar withdrawal.

Whatever happens, never, ever keep your favourite addictive foods (such as chocolate) in the home, not even for your children.

Have a treat every day. It should be something you like but are not normally addicted to. For instance, if you used to eat chocolate bars every day, replace them with home-made hot chocolate drinks. The 'comfort factor' won't be anything like 100 per cent at first, but after about two weeks it will reach the 80–90 per cent level. Commercial hot chocolate mixes are very high in sugar, so make your own by whisking cocoa powder and a little raw sugar into hot low-fat dairy milk or rice milk. Add a dash of vanilla for extra flavour. Every time you find yourself craving chocolate, take your mind off it by going to make yourself one of these drinks. Or eat a bowl of soup!

If you have consumed a lot of sugary foods and drinks in the recent past, you should take a good quality daily multivitamin with minerals (including chromium). This will help restore and rebalance your system and give your hormones the best chance of maintaining your blood sugar on an even keel, which will help control physical craving sensations.

addiction, not everyone finds it possible to cut down or stop eating comfort foods straight away, even if they follow a diet that leaves them never feeling hungry.

Food addictions can be as difficult to overcome as addictions to alcohol, tobacco and drugs. Chemical changes – perhaps the release of endorphins – occur in your body on eating the addictive food. These changes are experienced as pleasurable and comforting sensations, and the addiction comes from associating the food with these sensations. You can even begin to feel mildly depressed when the pleasant sensations wear off, and this can cause insatiable cravings that keep you eating the problem food, just as nicotine withdrawal symptoms – no matter how mild – keep people smoking.

Since most addictive foods are high in sugar, the depression may be due to the strong dip in blood sugar that occurs in some people a few hours after eating sugary foods. Eating or drinking something sweet provides an instant boost, but it starts the vicious circle all over again. A deficiency of the mineral chromium substantially aggravates blood sugar problems. Chromium is mostly found in whole-grain foods and gets very depleted when you consume a lot of sugary foods and drinks.

EXERCISE

The more accustomed your body gets to hard exercise, the faster your cells will use up and burn calories. But your cells do not just step up their metabolism during the period of exercise itself. Your metabolic rate remains high for up to 15 hours afterwards – so your calories will be burned up faster even while you are asleep.

To help you lose weight, exercise must be regular, and hard enough to make you sweat or breathe faster for at least 20 minutes, about three times a week. Examples are weight or circuit training, hill-walking, jogging, swimming and aerobics. You should also walk briskly or cycle whenever you can, use stairs instead of lifts and elevators, walk up escalators, do the housework twice as fast, and go dancing instead of sitting in pubs and bars. Try to park your car a few minutes' walk from where you're going. All these things make a difference.

Experts in physiology have known for years that a body with more lean tissue (also known as muscle) makes for a more rapid metabolic rate. But both men and women start to lose muscle in their 20s, which is why, by middle age, it can be so hard to lose weight. Muscle can only be regained by exercising. In a study carried out by Tufts University, eight men and four women aged 56 to 80 carried out strength-building exercises for 30 minutes three times a week for 12 weeks. This boosted their resting metabolic rate by an amazing eight per cent, and they had to consume an extra 300 calories a day to keep their body weight at the same level. Their muscles did not grow any larger on this programme, but they did become stronger and more metabolically active.

Strength-building exercises involve sustaining a muscle's effort – holding the muscle in its position of maximum tension for as long as possible. Weight-lifting is the best-known but not the only form of strength-building exercise. The body's weight itself can be used to sustain maximum muscular effort – for instance in sit-up exercises which involve remaining in the stomach muscles' position of maximum effort for a count of 10.

Most people live within reasonable distance of a local health club with a gym. An instructor is always available to give a supervised training programme to meet personal requirements, and teach clients how to follow it.

Women please note that a few hours' strength-building a week is very unlikely to result in hard muscles! On the contrary, improving the lean-to-fat ratio gives a woman a great shape and makes her feel lighter and more energetic for the simple reason that her muscles will find it easier to carry her around.

Strength-building exercises are best combined with exercises designed to build cardiovascular fitness. You can tell roughly what your level of cardiovascular fitness is by how easily you get out of breath. Cycling, swimming, running, aerobics and rowing are all suitable forms, and it is surprising how quickly your fitness improves if you practise any of these a few times a week, even if only for 20 minutes.

If you find it hard to motivate yourself to exercise alone, try finding an exercise partner who agrees to meet up with you on a regular basis.

THE IMPORTANCE OF BREAKFAST

Some people try to lose weight by skipping breakfast, but this isn't a good idea. Breakfast stimulates your metabolism to wake up after an overnight fast. The speed of your metabolism determines how quickly you burn calories, so if you don't eat breakfast, your metabolism may remain at its night-time rate – slow!

Some people say they feel less hungry throughout the morning if they do skip breakfast. However, this is because several hormones are working to conserve your blood sugar and slow down your metabolism. The hunger you may have experienced after eating breakfast was probably caused by eating the wrong kind of breakfast. A bowl of cereal or toast and coffee for breakfast is mainly carbohydrate. It will raise your blood sugar levels quickly, but the faster they rise, the faster they will also fall and the sooner you will feel hungry again. On the other hand, if you eat a more substantial breakfast which includes more protein and a little good quality oil or fat, you should feel satisfied and energetic until shortly before lunchtime. On the Big Healthy Soup Diet you may find you need a little top-up mid-morning, but that doesn't matter; you can eat as often as you like as long as it's only soup!

SUPPLEMENTS TO AID WEIGHT-LOSS

Supplements of conjugated linoleic acid (CLA) – a substance found in dairy fat – have been found in clinical trials to help improve body composition. After dieting, the test subjects who were taking CLA supplements put weight back on mostly in the form of lean tissue, whereas the control subjects (those not taking CLA) put weight back on mostly in the form of body fat.

Another useful supplement is the amino acid carnitine. This regulates the rate at which the body burns fat. Your body makes carnitine from lysine and methionine, with the help of vitamin C and iron, but if you are not making the maximum amount which your body can use to aid fat-burning, it will do you no harm to get a little extra in the form of supplements.

As with all other supplements, CLA and carnitine should be taken in accordance with the directions on the product label.

POWER SOUPS TO AID WEIGHT-LOSS

Power food	What it does	Soup number
Aduki or adzuki beans	According to Oriental medicine, these are good for the kidneys and help to soak up dampness (aid the release of water retention)	Pre-cook and add to any suitable soup, e.g. 22, 23, 24, 30, 43, 49
Apples	Rich in pectin which aids fullness by absorbing up to 100 times its weight in water	1, 5, 14, 25
Avocado pears	Rich in beneficial oils and in vitamin B_6	2, 15
Dark red, blue and purple fruits (bilberries, blueberries, blackberries, black cherries, black grapes etc.)	Rich in flavonoids which help to prevent excess water flow from capillaries into body tissues. Also have an antihistamine effect, helping to prevent inflammation which causes water retention	3, 4
Broad beans	Aid the release of water retention	7, 25
Cabbage	Rich in pectin which aids fullness by absorbing up to 100 times its weight in water	8, 9, 10, 11, 12, 13, 44, 61
Cayenne (chilli) pepper	Creates warmth which helps to stimulate the metabolism and drive off water retention	11, 15, 17, 30, 37, 39, 45, 47, 49, 57, 59, 60, 61

Power food	What it does	Soup number
Celery	Rich in coumarin, which aids the breakdown of protein sediments that act as a focus of water retention in body tissues	7, 23, 43, 55, 57
Citrus peel (zest)	Rich in flavonoids which help to prevent excess water flow from capillaries into body tissues. Widely used in Chinese medicine to aid the release of water retention	1, 16, 29, 45, 47, 57
Cucumber	Helps to promote urination without having the harshness of diuretics	17
Flax oil	An ideal oil to add to soup just before serving (never use it for cooking as this damages it). Helps maintain fullness and, unlike most oils, it is rich in both types of essential polyunsaturated fatty acids	7, 25 or add one tablespoon to any soup
Garlic	Traditionally viewed as a warming food which helps to drive off water retention. Lowers cholesterol and helps maintain normal blood pressure	8, 9, 11, 12, 14, 28, 39, 43, 45, 47, 49, 50, 51, 55, 56, 57, 60
Ginger	Creates warmth which helps to stimulate the metabolism and drive off water retention	6, 8, 11, 25, 38, 44, 48, 49, 53, 60
Liver	Rich in many nutrients such as B-complex vitamins and chromium which help to stimulate the metabolism	8

Power food	What it does	Soup number
Onion	Traditionally viewed as a warming food which helps to drive off water retention. Also has antiviral properties	Most of the recipes contain onion
Parsley	Rich in coumarin, which aids the breakdown of protein sediments that act as a focus of water retention in body tissues	7, 20, 23, 27, 29, 38, 41, 43, 48, 52
Psyllium husks	Rich in mucilage fibre which aids fullness by absorbing up to 100 times its weight in water	39
Radishes	Contain raphanin which helps to regulate the thyroid gland which governs metabolism	25, 44, 60, 61
Seaweed	Rich in iodine, needed by the thyroid gland which governs metabolism. Also rich in mucilage which aids fullness by absorbing up to 100 times its weight in water	8, 21, 44
Shrimps	Aid metabolism and water release by boosting Yang energy	46, 60
Soy foods: soy milk, tofu, soy flour, soy sauce, miso	Reduce cholesterol and help to balance oestrogen, which in excess can encourage water retention	12, 33, 36, 39, 41, 44, 47, 51

SOUP DIET PROGRAMMES

The two soup diet programmes in this book have been devised for you depending on your needs. If you want to clean out your system, shed some water retention and start getting into a more healthy state, Programme 1: the four-day Mini-detox, is for you.

If, on the other hand, you have some weight to lose, you can go straight to Programme 2: the 10-day Big Healthy Soup Diet. (This starts off with the same four-day Mini-detox.) You can repeat the diet as often as you like until you have reached your target weight. Alternatively, after the 10 days just begin to sample the other delicious soup recipes in this book. They are all designed to help you shed pounds.

Programme 1: Mini-detox

This is designed to

- Cleanse and begin to regenerate your digestive system
- Balance your blood sugar
- Reduce stress on your adrenal glands
- Re-hydrate your blood after too much alcohol, tea and coffee – but at the same time release unhealthy water retention from your tissues
- Eliminate excess acidity caused by too much meat, fat and sugar
- Provide extra antioxidants to combat toxins
- Start off the fat-burning process

The most essential part of any detox diet is to consume plenty of liquid. While cold liquids can actually cool and slow down some people's metabolism, warm liquids and hot soup can energize you and provide all the special ingredients that help to clean out your system. Unlike most detox diets, this one provides protein in the form of nuts, tofu, beans and avocado, so it is also safe to follow for longer periods and can be repeated up to four times (a total of 16 days).

FOUR-DAY MINI-DETOX

Day 1		Day 3	
Breakfast	Apple, almond and cardamom soup with yoghurt (Soup No. 1)	*Breakfast*	Dried fruit soup with pecans (Soup No. 5)
Lunch	Water release soup (Soup No. 7)	*Lunch*	Water release soup (Soup No. 7)
Dinner	Cream of cauliflower soup (Soup No. 40)	*Dinner*	Spinach and French lentil soup (Soup No. 58)
Day 2		**Day 4**	
Breakfast	Baked fruit, cashew and cinnamon soup (Soup No. 3)	*Breakfast*	Avocado and banana soup with almonds and strawberries (Soup No. 2)
Lunch	Water release soup (Soup No. 7)	*Lunch*	Water release soup (Soup No. 7)
Dinner	Mexican bean and lime soup with tofu (Soup No. 47)	*Dinner*	Brussels butterbean bisque (Soup No. 35)

IMPORTANT

Since you should not eat any other foods during these four days, make extra quantities of soup to eat as snacks. But don't overload your stomach! Part of the detox process involves not giving your stomach so much food that it has difficulty digesting it. Never continue eating beyond the point of feeling satisfied. You should also drink plenty of plain water (2 litres/4 pints a day) to carry away the dissolved wastes in your blood. This water must be plain and unflavoured, otherwise it will have a reduced capacity to absorb wastes and toxins. In addition to plain water, you may also drink fresh fruit juice diluted with water, and the herbal teas listed in the box on page 25.

HERBAL TEAS FOR USE WITH
THE MINI-DETOX

Chamomile: Promotes good digestion and helps you sleep

Dandelion root coffee: Helps to drain wastes from the liver

Fennel: Promotes good digestion

Ginger: Aids digestion and warms the circulation

Ginseng: Boosts vitality in older women during and after the menopause

Peppermint: Aids the flow of bile and promotes good digestion

Sage: Helps to relax blood vessels and promote circulation

If you have a juice extractor, try making juices from a mixture of carrot, radish, broccoli stems and celery. Drinking a wine-glassful of this juice twice a day will help to rejuvenate your liver and aid the release of unhealthy water retention. You can flavour the mixture with lemon juice, which contains ingredients that help to dissolve gallstones. Whizz in some parsley for extra benefits. Better still, dilute the juice with a large glass of water and whisk in a level tablespoon of psyllium husks. Drinks made in this way will help to sweep out your intestines, where toxins can become embedded if you don't normally have regular bowel motions.

You can stop at the end of the four days if you feel you have achieved the desired results. But if you feel good on this detox it will do you no harm to continue for longer.

Detox effects

All detox diets have side-effects, and this one is no exception. Be especially prepared for a day or two of headaches caused by withdrawal from caffeine. You may also feel a little tired and nauseous. These symptoms should pass as your body adjusts.

THE 10-DAY BIG HEALTHY SOUP DIET

Days 1–4, as for four-day Mini-detox (see page 24)

Day 5		Day 7	
Breakfast	Apple, almond and cardamom soup with yoghurt (Soup No. 1)	*Breakfast*	Dried fruit soup with pecans (Soup No. 5)
Lunch	Brown lentil soup with roasted sweet peppers and apricots (Soup No. 34)	*Lunch*	Red lentil and chestnut soup (Soup No. 52)
Dinner	Spicy cabbage soup with cod and garlic (Soup No. 11)	*Dinner*	Carrot, chicken and sweetcorn spicy chowder (Soup No. 37)
Day 6		**Day 8**	
Breakfast	Baked fruit, cashew and cinnamon soup (Soup No. 3)	*Breakfast*	Avocado and banana soup with almonds and strawberries (Soup No. 2)
Lunch	Mung bean soup with garlic and ginger (Soup No. 49)	*Lunch*	Sweet potato and groundnut soup (Soup No. 59)
Dinner	Salmon and potato chunky chowder (Soup No. 53)	*Dinner*	Thai shrimp noodle soup (Soup No. 60)

Day 9		Day 10	
Breakfast	Apple, almond and cardamom soup with sheep's yoghurt (Soup No. 1)	*Breakfast*	Baked fruit, cashew and cinnamon soup (Soup No. 3)
Lunch	Italian tomato and parsley soup (Soup No. 23)	*Lunch*	Potato and walnut pesto soup with tofu (Soup No. 51)
Dinner	Butternut bisque with Cajun-style red mullet (Soup No. 36)	*Dinner*	Moroccan chickpea chorba (Soup No. 48)

IMPORTANT

During the 10 days, eat only soups as directed. If you feel hungry between meals, snack on soup, if necessary taking one or two vacuum flasks of hot soup to work with you, or a container of ready-made soup which you can heat up at work if you have a kitchen.

If you wish to carry on losing weight after the 10 days, just continue on a soup-only diet, using the recipes in this book. Provided that you eat a soup from either the 'Cabbage Soups' or the 'Substantial Soups' sections at least once a day, you should not go short of protein. (Alternatively, to protein-enrich any of the soups in the 'Starters' section, add a portion of tofu or some poached fish or chicken.)

Since cow's milk products can cause water retention in some individuals, select the 'soy milk' and 'soy cream' options where they are offered as an alternative. If you appear to lose a lot of water retention during the 10 days of this programme, you will need to test yourself to find out which foods could be involved. *Waterfall Diet* publications (see Resources, page 277) are specifically designed to help you do this.

Programme 2: The 10-day Big Healthy Soup Diet

This is designed for longer-term weight loss. It starts with the four-day detox and continues with a further six days of soups to warm your metabolism and help you continue shedding water retention. If you do suffer from water retention, this common problem can easily add 8 lbs to your weight. So you could lose 2 lbs of fat and as much as 8 lbs of retained water by the end of the 10-day programme. That's a total of 10 lbs!

OTHER WAYS TO DIET WITH SOUP

Research shows that starting a meal with hot soup helps you to reduce the amount of food subsequently eaten. So if you find a soup-only diet a bit too difficult, you can start any meal with a bowl of soup, and you should feel satisfied much more easily. You could also try an occasional 'soup-only day'.

As you will see from the research at the end of this chapter, you cannot get the 'soup effect' just by drinking a beverage with solid food. The body seems to be able to tell the difference between liquid that is consumed separately, and liquid which forms part of the food itself.

MAINTAINING YOUR IDEAL WEIGHT

Reaching your target weight is often not the biggest problem with weight control: keeping it is. Yo-yo dieting is common, and is caused by relaxing your eating habits too much for too long once you have got rid of the excess pounds. We are all guilty of throwing caution to the winds after weeks or months of deprivation, and indulging in some 'well-deserved' binges. The problem is that we enjoy the binges so much that we can't stop them, and all our old habits creep back again! After reaching your target weight it really is important to be especially vigilant. If you are longing to binge, then by all means do so, but set yourself a programme and ration your high-calorie binge foods on a weekly basis. Decide in advance how many treats you will buy per week and when you will eat them. Whatever happens, *do not keep treats in the home*. Even if the treats are for other members of your family, you must make sure that they are not available to you at times when you are not allowed to eat them, as you will be far too tempted to raid the cookie jar when you are a little bit bored, depressed or peckish. The only safe way to ration treats is to buy them as and when you are allowed to eat them, in the exact quantities you are allowed.

Another pitfall is to promise yourself that you will make up for unscheduled binges at a later date. Believe me, you won't! The reason why you got overweight in the first place is that your favourite foods (usually sugar-rich foods) were just too addictive. Addictive behaviour is a slippery slope, and few people recognize it in themselves. If you understand this right at the start, you will have a better chance of keeping your beautiful new figure.

Soup is a fantastic aid to keeping your target weight. To help maintain your ability to resist snacking between meals, just continue to start each meal with a bowl of soup.

SKIN HEALTH

I have already mentioned that eating too many foods high in visible and especially invisible fats plays havoc with your skin (see page 6). Not only do pores get clogged, but blackheads form and greasiness develops. Fat slows down your blood circulation, and this reduces the supply of vitamins and oxygen to cells that make collagen. These cells may lose their efficiency and slow down collagen production. The less collagen you make, the more likely is the appearance of premature ageing. Not only does the Big Healthy Soup Diet have a carefully controlled fat and oil content, it is also very rich in nutrients which nourish your skin cells.

Dehydration from drinking too much tea, coffee and alcohol also harms your skin. Another benefit of soup is to give you plenty of liquid to help hydrate you.

Rich in dietary fibre, the Big Healthy Soup Diet also encourages regular, healthy bowel motions. This helps you eliminate toxins and soluble wastes, which could otherwise be absorbed from your intestines into your blood. Such toxins overload your kidneys and cause the typical sallow complexion of people who suffer from long-term constipation.

AMAZING DISCOVERIES ABOUT SOUP

2005 Study at Purdue University, Lafayette, USA

Solid and liquefied versions of identical foods high in protein, fat or carbohydrate (containing the same number of calories) were given to 13 male and 18 female volunteers. Beverages were also tested. The participants completed questionnaires on mood, appetite and psychological state. Eating soup led to reduced hunger. Overall calorie consumption tended to be lower on days when soup was eaten compared with days on solid foods and beverages. Beverages had the least effect on hunger reduction. The researchers concluded that soup may help to reduce appetite.

Mattes R. *Physiol Behav.* 2005 Jan 17;83(5):739–47.

2003 Study at the New York Obesity Research Center, St. Luke's-Roosevelt Hospital Center, New York, USA

Cholecystokinin (CCK) is a gut hormone that plays a role in satiety (feeling full). Levels of CCK rise after a meal, and this helps us to feel full. The researchers wanted to test whether soup quenches appetite by stimulating higher levels of CCK. They measured plasma CCK levels in eight healthy, non-obese men and women before and after eating 800 grams of tomato soup, followed 30 minutes later by 300 grams of a yoghurt shake. Appetite ratings were compared with CCK levels. It was found that eating soup significantly increased plasma CCK levels within 30 minutes in all subjects combined. Interestingly, the women's average CCK levels were significantly higher than the men's. The researchers concluded that eating soup may be especially beneficial for women who want to lose weight.

Nolan L.J. and colleagues. *Nutrition.* 2003 Jun;19(6):553–7.

1999 Research at the Pennsylvania State University, USA

Research has shown that adding water to foods can lead to reductions in the number of calories consumed. This study aimed to find out how water affected appetite when served separately with food or incorporated into food. Seventeen minutes before lunch, 24 women were fed one of three starters: (a) chicken-rice casserole, (b) chicken-rice casserole served with a glass of water, (c) chicken-rice soup. All the starters contained the same number of calories. The soup contained the same ingredients (type and amount) as the casserole that was served with water. The researchers found that turning the casserole into soup by adding water to it greatly increased fullness and reduced hunger. The equivalent amount of water served in a glass with the food did not aid fullness. Calorie intake at lunch was much less after the soup compared with after the casserole, whether water was served with the casserole or not. The test subjects did not compensate at dinner for eating less lunch.

Rolls B.J. and colleagues. *Am J Clin Nutr.* 1999 Oct;70(4):448–55.

1998 Study at the Nutritional Neurobiology Laboratory, EPHE, Paris, France

Twelve lean and ten overweight young men were given a starter consisting of (a) vegetables and water, or (b) puréed and strained vegetable soup, or (c) chunky vegetable soup. The soups were of the same composition and volume; only the size of the solid pieces and the distribution of nutrients between solids and liquid were different. All the starters were found to reduce hunger and subsequent food intake, but the chunky soup had the most pronounced effect. The researchers concluded that there may be special benefits in using chunky soups as part of a weight-loss programme.

Himaya A. and colleagues. *Appetite.* 1998 Apr;30(2):199–210.

1994 Study at the Centre for Human Nutrition, University of Sheffield, UK

The consumption of dietary fibre is known to prolong the feeling of fullness, but it was not known how. In this study on eight male volunteers, three per cent guar gum (a type of mucilage fibre similar to psyllium husks) was added to high-fat and low-fat soups. Guar gum delayed the emptying of the stomach for both types of soup, but the delays in the return of hunger and decline of fullness were far greater for the fatty soup. The fibre appeared to work by slowing absorption and prolonging the presence of nutrients in the intestines.

French S.J. and colleagues. *Am J Clin Nutr.* 1994 Jan;59(1):87–91.

1990 Study at Johns Hopkins University School of Medicine, Baltimore, USA

Three different starters – tomato soup, melon or cheese on crackers, all with the same number of calories – were served just before the main course. Soup was found to reduce the amount of food eaten in the second course much more than the other starters. The researchers concluded that eating soup could be beneficial in weight-reduction programmes.

Rolls B.J. and colleagues. *Appetite.* 1990 Oct;15(2):115–26.

PART II

STAYING HEALTHY
WITH SOUP

We all know that you are what you eat, and how important it is to eat vegetables. But that's not always as easy as it sounds. Some people find vegetables too bland, and children may refuse them altogether. But do you know anyone who doesn't like soup? Soup can help you and your loved ones reach a ripe old age without too many visits to the doctor. A single portion of soup can hold a lot of power foods which protect you with antioxidants, flavonoids, essential fatty acids and dietary fibre. For instance, a soup made with tomatoes, beans, garlic, onions, parsley and shredded dark green leaves (cabbages, collards or spring greens, Brussels tops etc.) can:

- Help to prevent heart disease and cancers (tomatoes, parsley, green leaves)
- Lower cholesterol (beans and garlic)
- Fight viruses (onions)

As regards preparing such a soup, the only limit is your imagination!

- Add lemon juice if you like your soup tart and zingy
- Or some Tabasco sauce or cayenne pepper if you prefer it spicy
- Or purée the soup and add a teaspoon of cream and some Parmesan cheese

Can something so delicious really prevent ill-health? Don't take my word for it; have a look at the research summaries at the end of this chapter (page 46). They are just a few examples of the many scientific studies that prove the tremendous health benefits of eating fruit and vegetables. They're so much easier to eat when you make them into soup! All the studies come to the same conclusion: the more fresh fruit and vegetables you eat, the less likely you are to get clogged arteries, high blood pressure, heart attacks and cancers. It's as straightforward as that. Once we had to take it all on trust that these major health problems (and the disabilities they bring) were food-related. Now it is no longer just naturopaths and alternative medicine specialists who are telling us these things, but doctors and scientists as well.

Next we need to ask 'How much is enough?' When I mention green vegetables, for instance, so many people say 'I do eat greens so I must be okay.' Then I discover they last ate them several weeks ago. This is actually a low frequency and puts the person in a high disease-risk category. If you really want these power foods to protect you, consider eating them every day. As you can see from the summaries on page 46, researchers recommend consuming 400–600 grams (1–1½ lbs) of fruit and vegetables per day. It's so easy when you add them to soup!

Good soups to start with are Soup 1: Apple, almond and cardamom soup with sheep's yoghurt, Soup 13: Traditional Ukrainian borscht, and Soup 34: Brown lentil soup with roasted sweet peppers and apricots. Or just work your way through the whole book to discover your favourite recipes, and put them on your daily menu!

POWER SOUPS FOR STAYING HEALTHY

Power food	Details	May help to prevent	Soup number
Apples	Rich in pectin, which helps to carry away traces of toxic metals in your intestinal contents	Kidney problems related to toxicity	1, 5, 14, 25
Beans, lentils	Rich in soluble fibre, B-vitamins, zinc. Help to slow down absorption of starches eaten in the same meal	Heart disease, blood sugar problems	7, 9, 25, 30, 34, 35, 40, 43, 45, 47, 49, 52, 58
Broccoli, cabbage, cauliflower, Brussels sprouts, watercress	Contain indoles which help your liver to break down chemicals and 'used' hormones	Breast cancer, ovarian cysts, endometriosis	8, 9, 10, 11, 12, 13, 32, 33, 35, 40, 44, 61
Dark red, blue and purple fruits (bilberries, blueberries, blackberries, black cherries, black grapes etc.)	Rich in antioxidants and flavonoids which fight inflammation. Natural antihistamine properties. Help the circulation in small blood vessels, especially in brain, eyes and ears	Arthritis, asthma, water retention, eye and ear problems, memory loss	3, 4
Brown rice	Rich in B-complex vitamins	Nervous problems	8, 11, 23, 24, 29, 37, 50

Power food	Details	May help to prevent	Soup number
Carrots	Rich in beta-carotene, the antioxidant precursor to vitamin A	Cancers, heart disease, eye problems	8, 13, 24, 27, 42
Cayenne	Warms the circulation, improving the microcirculation in the brain, eyes and ears	Circulatory problems	11, 15, 17, 30, 37, 39, 45, 47, 49, 57, 59, 60, 61
Celery	Rich in coumarin	Water retention, arthritis	7, 23, 43, 55, 57
Citrus peel and zest	Rich in flavonoids	Circulatory problems, water retention, varicose veins	1, 16, 29, 45, 47, 57
Coconut oil	Source of lauric acid, which combats the herpes virus. Does not raise cholesterol like other hard fats	Chronic viral infections	6, 46, 61
Coriander leaf (cilantro)	Accelerates excretion of toxic metals such as mercury and lead	Kidney problems related to toxicity	47, 49, 59, 60, 61
Cranberries	These help prevent bacteria adhering to bladder walls	Cystitis	Can be added to fruit soup recipes
Cucumber	Soothing for the urinary system	Cystitis	17

Power food	Details	May help to prevent	Soup number
Fenugreek seeds	Ground up, can help to soothe the digestive system	Digestive problems	30, 52
Fish and seafood	Rich in protein, zinc, iodine. Oily fish also provide essential polyunsaturated fatty acids	Heart disease and cancers	11, 36, 46, 53, 54, 55, 57, 60
Garlic	When raw, has many anti-infective properties, especially for the intestines and lungs	Parasitic diseases, AIDS, candidiasis, dysentery, food poisoning, worms, bronchitis	8, 9, 11, 12, 14, 28, 39, 43, 45, 47, 49, 50, 51, 55, 56, 57, 60
Ginger	Like cayenne, warms the circulation, especially in the digestive system	Circulatory problems, poor digestion	6, 8, 11, 25, 38, 44, 48, 49, 53, 60
Leafy greens	Rich in calcium, magnesium and many antioxidants	Blindness, cancers, heart disease, osteoporosis, nervous problems	7, 8, 9, 10, 11, 12, 13, 19, 23, 32, 44, 58, 60, 61
Mint	Acts as a balm for the digestive system and stimulates the flow of bile	Flatulence, gallstones	48

Power food	Details	May help to prevent	Soup number
Nuts, sunflower seeds, sesame seeds	Rich in the minerals magnesium and zinc, rich in the amino acid arginine, rich in essential polyunsaturated oils	Circulatory problems, high blood pressure, nervous problems	1, 2, 3, 5, 7, 14, 49, 51
Olive oil (extra-virgin)	Rich in the antioxidant squalene	Heart disease	Most of our recipes contain olive oil
Onions	Stimulate the flow of bile. Antiviral properties. Reduce cholesterol. Natural antihistamine properties	Chronic virus infections, high cholesterol, gallstones	Most of our recipes contain onion
Parsley leaf	Rich in vanadium and coumarin	Diabetes, water retention	7, 20, 23, 27, 29, 38, 41, 43, 48, 52
Pumpkin seeds	Rich in zinc and essential polyunsaturated oils. Contain an ingredient that combats prostate gland enlargement	Enlarged prostate	26
Radishes	Dry up the common cold, stimulate bile flow, contain raphanin which regulates thyroxine production by the thyroid gland	Gallstones, hypothyroidism, hyperthyroidism	25, 44, 60, 61

Power food	Details	May help to prevent	Soup number
Seaweed (e.g. nori, wakame, laverbread, arame)	Rich in iodine, which is needed to maintain normal levels of female hormones and thyroid hormone	Breast cancer, endometriosis, hypothyroidism	8, 21, 44
Soy foods: soy milk, tofu, soy flour, soy sauce, miso	Help to balance oestrogen. Work against prostate cancer. Lower cholesterol	Breast cancer, endometriosis, prostate cancer, heart disease	12, 33, 36, 39, 41, 44, 47, 51
Tomatoes	Rich in lycopene	Breast cancer, prostate cancer	8, 15, 17, 23, 26, 28, 43, 47, 57
Turmeric	Contains powerful antioxidant curcumin	Arthritis, liver problems, cancers	8, 30, 45, 48
Yoghurt	Live yoghurt contains living 'friendly' bacteria	Eaten regularly, helps to prevent bowel cancer and is a good remedy for travellers' diarrhoea	1, 2, 4, 5, 6, 34

Of course if you smoke, take no exercise, eat too much salty, fatty or sugary food and drink too much alcohol, then it is much harder for good foods to protect you. After all, no matter how much good quality engine oil you put in your car, it will still break down if you put the wrong fuel in the tank!

FOODS THAT NEED TO BE RATIONED

Food	Health effects
Alcohol	Stresses your liver and dehydrates you. Promotes several cancers.
Artificial food additives	These are added in large amounts to yoghurt and soft drinks, sweets and convenience foods. Some are sold as sugar substitutes to add to tea and coffee etc. Some sweeteners are linked with headaches, dizziness and epilepsy. Many children develop behavioural symptoms on exposure to colourings. Some preservatives are linked with asthma. Potential harmful health effects of combining different additives have not been researched and are unknown.
Bad fats	These are mainly hydrogenated fats and other highly processed fats hidden in margarine, cakes, pastries, biscuits, cookies and other convenience foods. These encourage high cholesterol and clogged arteries, and prevent your body from using essential polyunsaturated oils. Excess consumption of animal fats also encourages high cholesterol.
Deep-fried foods	These are a separate issue from high-fat foods because not only are they high in fat, they also have other harmful effects on health. At the prolonged high temperatures of deep-frying, chemical changes such as peroxidation take place at great speed. A high intake of fried foods is directly associated with a higher risk of several cancers. In one study, women with a pre-cancerous condition of the breast showed signs of being heavier consumers of deep-fried foods than other women. The highest risk of colon cancer is linked with the frequent intake of meat which has been fried or grilled until charred or heavily browned.

Food	Health effects
Eggs	Eaten in moderation, eggs are a good, healthy food. But because they are hard to digest, people with a weak digestion can more easily become intolerant ('allergic') to them, leading to problems such as migraine and arthritis.
Gluten and cow's milk protein	Like eggs, these are hard to digest. There is increasing evidence that eating too much gluten (found mainly in wheat) promotes gluten deposits in tissues, which then become a focus for chronic inflammation and auto-immunity (see page 72). The same can apply to cow's milk proteins. Ceasing to eat these items has been found to improve many chronic health problems, including arthritis, migraine and even childhood autism. To avoid a build-up of gluten deposits, it is best to eat pasta, bread and other baked goods only a few times a week rather than several times a day, which is the custom in the West.
Salt and sodium (the main component of salt)	A high salt (sodium) intake has been linked with water retention, high blood pressure and weight gain (as a result of water retention), osteoporosis and asthma. Again, much of our salt intake is hidden in foods such as salami, ham and bacon, sausages, smoked fish, canned foods, salty cheeses, salted nuts, crisps (potato chips) and other packet snacks, bread, stock cubes, yeast extract, soy sauce and ready-prepared pies, pastries, sauces, or commercially manufactured 'oven-ready' dishes. Most commercial soft drinks are very high in sodium. Baking powder and some medicines, such as antacids based on bicarbonate of soda or effervescent tablets of any kind, also contain large amounts of sodium. One of the most common food additives is a flavour-enhancer known as monosodium glutamate or 'E621'.

Food	Health effects
Soft drinks	These are colas and similar carbonated drinks in cans or bottles. They contain large amounts of artificial colouring and flavouring, plus either sugar or artificial sweeteners. A can of cola can contain up to 10 lumps of sugar. Some people get so hooked on these drinks that they feel ill if deprived for just one day. Due to the artificial sweeteners, drinking the 'diet' varieties can lead to headaches and dizziness – and in extreme cases even ear and brain problems. These drinks usually have a high phosphorus content, which stimulates calcium losses from our bones.
Sugar	Added sugar – and this includes honey and syrup, which are also concentrated sugar – is absorbed very fast, making your insulin rise too quickly and too high. Scientific trials show that high insulin encourages high fat levels in your blood, and cholesterol deposits on your artery walls. Your blood also becomes more 'sticky', and so prone to tiny clots that could lead to a heart attack as you get older. High insulin levels make you gain weight: you retain sodium, which encourages water retention, and you form body fat more easily, especially around your middle. Eventually the body can develop a resistance to insulin, and this condition leads to diabetes. Most added sugar is 'hidden' in cakes, cookies, biscuits, chocolate, sweets, desserts, ice cream, soft drinks, tea and coffee. In the UK, the average sugar consumption is about one kilo or two pounds a week. This is far too much for us to expect to remain in good health.

Food	Health effects
Tea and coffee	These have a diuretic effect. They make you urinate more, which encourages dehydration, increased losses of magnesium and other minerals, and also makes your kidneys retain sodium. Dehydration increases the risk of arthritis, since joints become more easily worn when their water content is reduced. Taken with meals, tea and coffee substantially reduce the absorption of iron and zinc from your food. This may account for why some researchers believe these drinks can encourage infertility. Coffee is a nervous system stimulant which may provoke anxiety and panic attacks in susceptible people. It also increases your liver's workload.

Don't be dismayed at this long list. Of course you can still be healthy without giving up all these foods! Some people even feel guilty if they buy butter for their children and eat some of it themselves. That is a natural reaction, but it is actually a huge over-reaction. Rationing is recommended – total deprivation is not! I eat most of these foods myself, but as occasional treats rather than as staple parts of my daily diet.

The easiest way to ration is to consume so much of the right foods that you don't feel as much need for the wrong ones. If you have a big problem with craving sweets, chips, fries and pastries, try eating a bowl of home-made soup first. It is one of the best ways to take the edge off cravings.

WE DO NEED TO EAT SOME SUGAR EVERY DAY, DON'T WE?

This is not at all true as all the carbohydrate you eat gets turned into sugar by your body. If you still need more you can turn protein and parts of the fat molecule into sugar. To get enough energy there's no need to consume any sugar or sugary foods at all.

AMAZING FOOD AND HEALTH DISCOVERIES

2003 Article from the Division of Preventive Medicine, Harvard Medical School, Boston, Massachusetts, USA

Heart disease is still the leading cause of disease and death worldwide. Statistics show that populations who consume more fruits and vegetables often have a lower risk of developing heart disease, high blood pressure and diabetes. Recent large research studies show that the higher the fruit and vegetable intake, the lower the rate of heart attacks and strokes. Many nutrients in fruits and vegetables, including fibre, potassium and folic acid, help to reduce the risk. The low glycaemic index and calorie content of these foods may also play a part. In view of these benefits, the researchers believe that not enough effort and resources are currently being devoted to encouraging dietary changes in Western society.

Bazzano L.A., Serdula M.K., Liu S. *Curr Atheroscler Rep.* 2003 Nov;5(6):492–9.

2004 Article from the UCLA Center for Human Nutrition, Los Angeles, USA

An intake of 400–600 grams (1– 1¹/₂ lbs) of fruits and vegetables per day brings lower rates of many common forms of cancer. Diets rich in plant foods also bring a lower risk of heart disease and chronic diseases of ageing. Red foods such as tomatoes contain lycopene, which has special benefits for prostate health. Green foods, including broccoli, Brussels sprouts and kale, contain glucosinolates, which protect against cancer. Garlic and other foods in the onion family contain allyl sulphides which may inhibit cancer cell growth. Substances in green tea and soybeans also have health benefits. Everyone would potentially benefit from consuming one serving of each of the seven colour groups daily. The United States National Cancer Institute and American Institute for Cancer Research already recommend five to nine servings of fruit and vegetables per day.

Heber D. *J Postgrad Med.* 2004 Apr–Jun;50(2):145–9.

2004 Article from the Department of Cardiology, All India Institute of Medical Sciences, New Delhi, India

The role of diet and nutrition in heart disease and stroke has been extensively researched. Enough evidence is available from population studies to show that the right diet can reduce the risk of heart disease. Trans-fats and saturated fats increase the risk, while polyunsaturated fats are protective. Sodium raises the blood pressure, while foods rich in potassium reduce the risk of high blood pressure and stroke. Regular frequent consumption of fruits and vegetables protects against high blood pressure, heart attack and stroke. It is time to translate this knowledge into government policies that promote healthy diets and discourage unhealthy diets.

Srinath Reddy K., Katan M.B. *Public Health Nutr.* 2004 Feb;7(1A):167–86.

1994 Article from Loma Linda University, California, USA

Recent research shows that frequent consumption of nuts offers protection against heart attacks. Nuts help to lower cholesterol, and also contain nutrients which protect in other ways.

Sabate J., Fraser G.E. *Curr Opin Lipidol.* 1994 Feb;5(1):11–6.

2004 Research Study from the London School of Hygiene and Tropical Medicine, UK

South Asian women from India eat a diet rich in phyto- (plant) oestrogens – not from soy foods but from beans, lentils and vegetables. The dietary intake of phyto-oestrogens was compared between 240 South Asian women living in England with breast cancer, and 477 similar women without breast cancer. It was found that among the women with the highest intake of phyto-oestrogens there were only half as many cases of breast cancer as among those with the lowest intake. The researchers concluded that phyto-oestrogens help to protect against breast cancer.

dos Santos Silva I., Mangtani P. and colleagues. *Cancer Causes Control.* 2004 Oct;15(8):805–18.

2004 Article from the Hallelujah Acres Foundation, Ellensburg, Washington, USA

Scientists estimate that 30–40 per cent of all cancers can be prevented by lifestyle and dietary measures alone. Consuming too much low-fibre food and red meat, and a poor balance of essential polyunsaturated fats, increases the risk of developing cancer. Consuming abundant fruits and vegetables lowers cancer risk. Garlic, onions and cruciferous vegetables such as broccoli and Brussels sprouts are especially beneficial. Nutrients that protect against cancer include selenium, folic acid, vitamin B_{12}, vitamin D, chlorophyll, and antioxidants such as carotenoids. Taking supplements of digestive enzymes and probiotics is also helpful. Individuals who follow these guidelines are likely to have a 60–70 per cent lower risk of developing breast, colon or prostate cancer, and also a reduced risk of contracting other forms of cancer.

Donaldson M.S. *Nutr J*. 2004 Oct 20;3(1):19.

2005 Research from the American Cancer Society, Atlanta, Georgia, USA

In this study, 148,610 adults aged 50–74 were asked to provide information on their consumption of meat in 1982 and again in 1992. They were observed from 1992 to 2001 and, during this time, 1,667 of them developed cancer of the colon or rectum (colorectal cancer). Those with colorectal cancer were found to be the highest long-term consumers of red meat and processed meats. The researchers concluded that prolonged high consumption of red meat and processed meats may increase the risk of cancer in the lower part of the large intestine. These findings have also been confirmed by other researchers.

Chao A., Thun M.J. and colleagues. *JAMA*. 2005 Jan 12;293(2):172–82.

2004 Research from Clemson University, SC, USA

Plants are known to contain anti-cancer compounds. The initial step in the formation of a cancer is damage to a cell, which leads to a mutation in one of its genes. Fresh juices and extracts from strawberries, raspberries and blueberries were evaluated for their ability to inhibit mutations induced by mutagens such as benzopyrene – a mutagen found in charred meat. The researchers found that juice from strawberries, raspberries and blueberries significantly inhibited the action of mutagens.

Hope Smith S., Tate P.L. and colleagues. *J Med Food.* 2004 Winter;7(4):450–5.

2004 Research from Michigan State University, USA

Anthocyanidins are pigments found in bilberries, blueberries, black grapes and other dark blue, dark red and purple fruits. On testing, these researchers found that they have a significant anti-cancer effect.

Zhang Y., Vareed S.K., Nair M.G. *Life Sci.* 2005 Feb 11;76(13):1465–72. Epub 2004 Dec 13.

1997 Research from Andrews University, Michigan, USA

A diet rich in plant foods contains many substances with health-protective benefits. Nuts, whole grains, fruit and vegetables contain phenolic compounds, terpenoids, pigments and other natural antioxidants that help to protect against and/or treat chronic diseases such as heart disease, cancer, diabetes and high blood pressure. The foods and herbs with the highest anti-cancer activity include garlic, soybeans, cabbage, ginger, liquorice, and cruciferous vegetables such as broccoli and cabbage. The phytochemicals in whole grains reduce the risk of heart disease and cancer. In addition to providing an ample supply of vitamin C, folic acid, potassium and pectin, citrus fruits also contain a host of active phytochemicals.

Craig W.J. *J Am Diet Assoc.* 1997 Oct;97(10 Suppl 2):S199–204.

PART III

FEELING GOOD
WITH SOUP

As we get older, the vitality of our digestive system often decreases. Food is less easily digested, absorbed and assimilated into cells. Your whole body is made from cells. While the vitamin and mineral levels in our food remain the same, amounts of nutrients getting into our cells may decrease. Depending on which types of cells are affected, problems can start to develop with hormones, energy, bones, joints, nervous system, immune system or circulation. These problems are often put down to the ageing process. But the good news is that ageing cells can be rejuvenated.

Cells are very much like miniature plants. Give them enough oxygen and nutrients, and help them to get rid of their waste products quickly, and they will be able to regenerate themselves and work more efficiently. The result is better energy, more balanced hormones, stronger bones and joints, and a healthier circulation and nervous system.

If by now you're guessing that the best way to rejuvenate your body is with soup, you are not far wrong. With less efficient digestion and absorption, it's important to reduce the load on your digestive system while increasing the nutrient density of what you eat. That means eating foods with a high ratio of vitamins, minerals and flavonoids compared with the total number of calories.

The most high-calorie foods are those high in sugar, fat and starch. Soup, on the other hand, quickly fills you up without containing added sugar, and with only a little fat (oil) and starch in the form of rice or potatoes. The rest is water, fibre, vitamins, minerals and protein. The fibre content helps to sweep out wastes which might otherwise be absorbed into your blood and end up burdening your kidneys. All these qualities make home-made soup a naturally rejuvenating food.

To increase the nutritional value of soup even more, you can enrich it with juice extracted from vegetables such as broccoli stems, carrots, tomatoes, radishes and celery. Consumed on a regular basis, soup made in this way helps your brain, nervous system, liver, kidneys, circulation and glands to work better. With a healthy circulation, your memory, energy, eyes and ears stay youthful, helping you to continue enjoying life well into old age. Cells discharge their wastes more easily, water retention recedes, and all sorts of ailments begin to disappear. Add home-made chicken or fish stock or broth and you can even help to rebuild joints and cartilage. Stock from boiled chicken and fish bones is rich in glucosamine, which scientists have successfully used to treat long-term arthritis and other inflammatory conditions.

MEDICINAL FOODS

Countless other ingredients with medicinal effects can easily be added to soup in truly delicious combinations. Ranging from coriander leaf (cilantro) to ginger, radishes, garlic and Brussels sprouts, these mouth-watering ingredients will make you feel as if you are in a top-class restaurant rather than taking your medicine. In this section we will look at how different soups can treat as well as prevent problems relating to the following body systems:

- Energy
- Immune system and detoxification
- Circulation (including brain, nerves, eyes, ears)
- Bones and joints
- Hormones

If you are feeling sceptical, and believe that only powerful medicines can reverse health problems, think again. How many people do you know who are taking prescription medicines for long-term health conditions? Are they being cured? Prescription drugs can make you feel better while you are taking them; in fact some drugs, including those for high blood pressure, are essential for your own safety. But drugs do not usually cure long-term problems. If they did, the problems would not be long-term! Over many years, a combination of genetics, stress and faulty lifestyle silently changes a person's internal environment and body chemistry to produce ailments and ill-health. No drug has ever been able to reverse this process. Food and nutrition are the real key not only to preventing ill-health but also to reversing it.

There's plenty of scientific proof too, although it's widely scattered and the work is poorly funded. My book *Treat Yourself with Nutritional Therapy* (see Resources, page 277) lists hundreds of scientific research studies written up in many different scientific and medical journals ranging from the *Lancet* to the *American Journal of Clinical Nutrition*. Some doctors do pay attention to this research, and treat their patients using a nutritional approach. Some of the organizations to which these doctors belong are listed under Resources on page 277.

I'VE ALREADY CHANGED MY DIET FOR THE BETTER!

If you are still sceptical because you have already made some healthy changes to your diet without feeling any better, this could just mean that you haven't yet found the right changes you need to make. With so many books bombarding you with different opinions about nutrition, it has become a very confusing subject. Bear in mind also that curing a health problem requires a lot of extra effort compared with just preventing it. For instance, take one of my cases, whose name was Richard.

Richard packed shelves in a supermarket and was 32 years old. For eight years he had had what appeared to be a huge scab measuring about two inches in diameter on his slightly balding head.

Richard had consulted many doctors with this problem. 'They just dab at it with stuff and then send me away,' he said in desperation. 'They won't tell me what it is and nothing they've given me has ever stopped it.' His self-confidence had been destroyed by this problem. He confessed that he couldn't stop thinking about it and imagined that other people were always looking at the scab. He really wanted a girlfriend, but believed that no-one would want him with this unsightly problem.

Richard had worked hard at his diet. He had grown up on a diet of very ordinary food: 'meat and two veg', chips, fries, lots of sweet tea and coffee. He had never consumed excessive amounts of sweets, chocolates or soft drinks, and his saturated fat consumption was no higher than the average. In the last year he had made efforts to eat more vegetables and salads, and had given up most fried foods as well as biscuits, cookies and the occasional bar of chocolate. There was no improvement in his scalp condition.

I explained that like his doctors I did not know what could be causing his problem, but that skin conditions usually responded quite well to making more drastic dietary changes. These were often only required temporarily until the condition cleared up. Richard was prepared to go ahead and see what could be achieved on that basis.

I gave Richard a diet that completely excluded saturated fat, dairy products and red meat, which contain arachidonic acid, a pro-inflammatory substance found in animal fats. Arachidonic acid can also be made within the body, but if excluded from foods eaten in the diet, the overall body load will be decreased. The diet also excluded tea and coffee, artificial food additives and alcohol. I asked

Richard to make lots of home-made soups and to throw every vegetable he could think of into them. He did this with pleasure. I also asked him to take vitamin A and zinc supplements, and fish oils, plus some herbs which would help to rejuvenate his liver.

Nothing much seemed to happen for the first few weeks, then we noticed that as Richard's hair grew, the scab seemed to be gradually lifting off with it. By the 10th week it had grown out completely, and the skin underneath was normal.

Cases like this are not unusual. It seems so sad that more people don't realize just how much can be achieved with dietary therapy. Richard's confidence and sense of self-worth had been severely scarred by so many years of enduring this unsightly problem.

BOOSTING ENERGY
WITH SOUP

Energy problems can range from getting easily tired after exertion to feeling exhausted almost all the time, no matter how much rest you have had. (This extreme condition is known as chronic fatigue syndrome or CFS.)

An energy problem can stem from long-term faulty nutrition, or from simply taking on too much and feeling unable to cope. Depression also makes you feel as if you have an energy problem. Everything seems like too much effort, and you just want to lie around doing nothing. This is why doctors sometimes prescribe antidepressant drugs for chronic fatigue.

But drugs cannot cure conditions caused or aggravated by a shortage of nutrients. Many nutrients are involved in the body's energy production processes. The adrenal hormones and neurotransmitters which keep us feeling happy are also made from nutrients. These nutrients – which include several B-vitamins, zinc and magnesium – are found at comparatively low levels in the average modern diet of processed convenience foods and white flour.

If you are still sceptical and think that nutrition can't really make any difference to how energetic or happy you feel, just think about the condition known as anaemia. Anaemia occurs when a lack of iron, B-vitamins, zinc, magnesium or copper results in reduced oxygen levels in the blood. This causes depleted energy, which may be accompanied by breathlessness, apathy and other symptoms, and it does not go away until the deficiency is treated with appropriate dietary measures or supplementation.

It's not always easy for a doctor to spot borderline nutritional deficiencies. Some deficiencies don't show up in standard blood tests until they are very advanced and have probably been progressively getting worse for years. Modern, more sensitive tests are now available which can detect a deficiency at an earlier stage, but these tests are more expensive, and the trend is for doctors to assume your diet is okay and that you don't need them. If you would like to be tested, you will need to contact one of the practitioner organizations listed under Resources on page 278.

Chronic fatigue syndrome and its twin condition fibromyalgia (chronic fatigue accompanied by muscle pains) is becoming increasingly common. The research studies on page 64 suggest that there is a strong link between chronic fatigue or depression, and undetected nutritional deficiencies.

High-strength nutritional supplements are used in scientific research since they produce the clearest results. But if you are treating yourself at home, your first concern should be to get the maximum nourishment from your food. What better way to do this than with soup?

To help improve your energy, try to eat at least one bowl of soup a day containing one or more of the power foods listed in the table below. Good ones to start with are Soup 30: South Indian spicy sambhar soup, Soup 60: Thai shrimp noodle soup, and Soup 61: Thai chicken and vegetable soup.

POWER SOUPS FOR BETTER ENERGY

Power food	What it does	Soup number
Brazil nuts	A good source of selenium, which is important to prevent depression-related lack of energy. Also a good source of the amino acid methionine, which is important for healthy adrenal glands	2
Brown rice	Rich in B-complex vitamins, needed to process carbohydrates into energy	8, 11, 23, 24, 29, 37, 50
Buckwheat	Similar properties to brown rice	44
Cayenne (chilli) pepper	Warms the circulation and helps get oxygen and nutrients to the tissues	11, 15, 17, 30, 37, 39, 45, 47, 49, 57, 59, 60, 61
Cheese	A good source of tyrosine, which helps to make antidepressant adrenal and thyroid hormones	12, 19, 23, 33
Cinnamon, cloves, cardamom	Act as antiseptics in the intestines, inhibiting the growth of bacteria and fungi which create fatigue-producing toxins	1, 3, 5, 30
Coconut oil	Toxic to 'stealth' microbes, which lack a cell wall and so may go undetected by the immune system. Such microbes have been linked with chronic fatigue syndrome	6, 46, 61

Power food	What it does	Soup number
Coriander leaves (cilantro)	May be able to help rid the body of toxic metals such as mercury, which can contribute to chronic fatigue	47, 49, 59, 60, 61
Fish and seafood	A good source of selenium, which is important to prevent depression-related lack of energy	11, 36, 46, 53, 54, 55, 57, 60
Flax oil (cold-pressed)	Added after soup has been cooked, this helps to stabilize the mitochondrial membranes in your cells, where energy is produced	7, 25 or can be added to any of the recipes
Garlic	When raw, garlic acts as an antiseptic in the intestines, inhibiting the growth of bacteria and fungi known to create fatigue-producing toxins	8, 9, 11, 12, 14, 28, 39, 43, 45, 47, 49, 50, 51, 55, 56, 57, 60
Ginger	Warms the circulation in the digestive tract, helping the organs of digestion and absorption to work more efficiently. Also a good Yang tonic	6, 8, 11, 25, 38, 44, 48, 49, 53, 60
Leafy greens	Rich in magnesium, which is needed to turn carbohydrates into energy. Rich in folic acid, which is often deficient in depression-related lack of energy	7, 8, 9, 10, 11, 12, 13, 19, 23, 32, 44, 58, 60, 61
Olive oil	Inhibits the growth of fungi known to create fatigue-producing toxins	Most of our recipes contain olive oil

Power food	What it does	Soup number
Onion	When raw, onion is soothing and healing for the intestines. It has similar properties to raw garlic	Most of our recipes contain onion
Peanuts	A good source of tyrosine, which helps to make antidepressant adrenal and thyroid hormones	46, 59
Rosemary	A natural antidepressant with antibacterial and antifungal properties	26, 28
Shrimps	In Oriental medicine, considered to be a good energy booster because they are one of the best Yang tonics. Also rich in zinc	46, 60
Sunflower seeds	A good source of tryptophan, which helps to make the antidepressant neurotransmitter serotonin	7
Yoghurt	Contains 'friendly' bacteria that inhibit the growth of intestinal fungi known to create fatigue-producing toxins	1, 2, 4, 5, 6, 28, 34

AMAZING DISCOVERIES ABOUT ENERGY

2000 Research from the UCLA School of Medicine, California, USA

The published science on chronic fatigue suggests that marginal nutritional deficiencies may be partly to blame. These include deficiencies of various B-vitamins, vitamin C, magnesium, sodium, zinc, L-tryptophan, L-carnitine, coenzyme Q10 and essential fatty acids. The researcher recommends that individuals with chronic fatigue should be tested for deficiencies and treated where appropriate since continued deficiencies may delay their recovery.

Werbach M.R. *Altern Med Rev*. 2000 Apr;5(2):93–108.

1999 research from King's College School of Medicine, London, UK

Some patients with chronic fatigue say they benefit from taking vitamin supplements. These researchers assessed vitamins B_1, B_2 and B_6 levels in the blood and cells of 12 chronic fatigue patients compared with 18 healthy people. Levels of all three vitamins were found to be so low in the fatigue patients that they could not make proper amounts of important enzymes. Vitamin B_6 was found to be particularly low.

Heap L.C. and colleagues. *J R Soc Med*. 1999 Apr;92(4):183–5.

1993 Research from Addenbrooke's Hospital, Cambridge, UK

The researchers measured levels of the B-vitamin folic acid in 60 patients with chronic fatigue. Abnormally low levels were found in as many as 50 per cent of cases.

Jacobson W. and colleagues. *Neurology*. 1993 Dec;43(12):2645–7.

1994 Research Reported in the *Journal of Nutritional Medicine*

Patients suffering from depression have been found to have disturbances in their ability to metabolize the B-vitamin folic acid. The disturbances are caused by a lack of vitamin B_6, B_{12}, magnesium and zinc, and the depression improves when these deficiencies are treated.

Lietha R. and colleagues. *J Nutr Med*. 1994;4:441–447.

1989 Research from the Royal Liverpool Hospital, UK

Levels of folic acid were estimated in the serum of depressed patients and found to be significantly lower than in normal people. The lower the folic acid levels the more severe the depression.

Abou-Saleh M.T. and colleagues. *Acta Psychiatr Scand.* 1989;80(1):78–82.

2004 Research from the Imperial College School of Medicine, Hammersmith Hospital, London, UK

Some research suggests that fish oil therapy can help to treat chronic fatigue syndrome (CFS). A woman who had suffered from CFS for six years, and had an enlarged heart due to the disease, was given purified fish oil supplements to take for 16 weeks, and her progress was measured. Within six to eight weeks she felt a marked improvement in her symptoms. Her enlarged heart also reduced in size.

Puri B.K. and colleagues. *Int J Clin Pract.* 2004 Mar;58(3):297–9.

2002 Research from the Department of Psychology, University of Wales, Swansea, UK

Selenium is an essential trace element but the level of selenium in plant foods depends on the soil in which they are grown. Some countries have soil with very low selenium levels. Selenium seems to be especially important for brain function, and five studies have reported a connection between a low selenium intake and depression. When selenium levels are low, depression can be successfully treated with selenium supplementation.

Benton D. *Nutr Neurosci.* 2002 Dec;5(6):363–74.

1996 Research from the USDA-ARS Western Human Nutrition Research Center (WCH), San Francisco, California, USA

Eleven healthy men were given a selenium-rich or selenium-poor experimental diet for 99 days. Those who had a low selenium level to start with became significantly more depressed than the others.

Hawkes W.C. and colleagues. *Biol Psychiatry.* 1996;39(2):121–8.

1982 Research from the Department of Psychiatry, University of Arizona, Tucson, USA

The neurotransmitter noradrenaline, needed for mood balance, is made from the amino acid tyrosine. Some individuals can be successfully treated for depression with tyrosine supplements.

Gelenberg A.J. and colleagues. *J Psychiatr Res.* 1982;17(2):175–80.

1998 Research Reported in *Integrated Physiology and Behavioral Science*

An assessment was made of 50 people diagnosed with chronic fatigue syndrome or fibromyalgia who on their own account had been taking nutritional supplements including freeze-dried fruits and vegetables and a vitamin/mineral complex. All had received some form of medical treatment prior to taking the nutritional supplements, but none with success lasting more than a few months. Nutritional supplements led to a steady and significant reduction in symptom severity in the period between initial assessment and follow-up.

Dykman K.D. and colleagues. *Integr Physiol Behav Sci.* 1998 Jan–Mar;33(1):61–71.

SOUP FOR A HEALTHY
IMMUNE SYSTEM

We think of our immune system as our defence against colds and infections. We are aware, too, that our immune system is vulnerable and can become deficient, leading to serious infections such as pneumonia (common in elderly people), and in extreme cases to AIDS.

What most of us don't know about the immune system is that it is also capable of causing a wide range of health problems if it fails to switch itself off after doing its job. These are known as 'auto-immune' health problems, and they include rheumatoid arthritis, emphysema, kidney disease, Crohn's disease, multiple sclerosis and even Alzheimer's disease. Food can help to prevent both immune deficiency and auto-immunity.

So is there an 'immune-boosting' soup which, as winter approaches, will help to prevent colds? I've always been hesitant to talk about 'boosting' the immune system. It gives the impression that eating a certain food or taking a supplement can increase your protection. I think that's a bit misleading, because if you are eating the kind of nourishing diet your whole body needs, your immune system will already be performing at its best. Adding anything extra won't really make any difference.

VITAMIN C

The one possible exception is vitamin C. Along with guinea pigs, monkeys and one type of bat, humans belong to a very small group of mammals which seems to have lost its ability to make its own vitamin C within the liver. Apparently we have a whole chain of enzymes designed to do just that, but the very last enzyme in the chain is missing. That forces us to get all our vitamin C from food, and there has been a great deal of controversy about just how much vitamin C is enough.

The late Nobel laureate Linus Pauling thought it made sense for humans to eat as much vitamin C per day as a man-sized animal (e.g. a goat) would be able to make in its liver. This can go up to 12,000 milligrams a day in the case of infections or stressful situations. Monkeys, which, like humans, have to rely on food to supply their vitamin C, consume up to 3,500 mg in their natural daily diet. When you consider that an orange may contain only about 60 mg, and that many people don't even eat that much vitamin C-rich food every day, you can imagine what effect such a low intake could have on our immune system.

It is quite difficult to get 3,500 mg from food. In fact, you would need to consume the juice of about 58 oranges a day to ensure that your immune system gets the same amount of vitamin C as a monkey's. Alternatively, you could just eat a good quality diet and add a couple of daily vitamin C pills. Research studies (see page 76) show that this does in fact seem to boost the size and activity of white blood cells in humans.

Stimulating your blood circulation is also a good way to maximize the efficiency of your immune system. You can do this with exercise, cold showers and by adding ginger and cayenne (chilli) pepper to your food. These two spices encourage a good blood flow, which helps to supply nutrients and oxygen not only to your immune cells, but also to your brain, adrenal glands and so on. Cayenne and ginger are especially helpful for elderly people, and can improve their vitality in general.

OTHER NUTRIENTS

Apart from vitamin C, the strength of your immune system suffers if it does not get the recommended amounts of vitamin A, zinc, iron, vitamin B6 and protein. Selenium is also important. Research shows that when selenium is lacking, viruses proliferate more easily.

A lack of protein affects the immune system most seriously. In developing countries where good quality protein can be hard to get, millions of people are at risk of contracting life-threatening infections. There are many scientists and doctors who believe that most, if not all, African AIDS is caused by poverty and malnutrition rather than by a specific virus.

As you can see, the Jewish tradition of giving chicken soup to the sick makes a lot of sense. In poor European and Middle Eastern communities of days gone by it is quite likely that many families were not able to eat protein every day. No doubt some had to survive for long periods on little more than bread and potatoes. But they knew that protein was needed to fight sickness, so a precious chicken would be slaughtered and made into soup.

In the West we are luckier, and most of us eat too much protein rather than too little. But I have occasionally come across people who through ignorance have been living on very low-protein diets consisting of only salad leaves and vegetables, sometimes in the mistaken belief that this is a healthy diet which can be safely followed for months or years. On the contrary, a severe lack of protein leads to water retention and problems with weight-loss.

AUTO-IMMUNITY

Our body is designed to stop foreign particles such as bacteria and bits of undigested gluten from entering our bloodstream. If it does not succeed, however, then antibodies from our immune system attach themselves to the particles, to form circulating immune complexes (CICs). These attract white cells called macrophages to swallow them up, thus destroying the foreign particles. Activated macrophages produce chemicals called cytokines, which tell the immune system to go into inflammatory mode. Inflammatory mode is characterized by heat, swelling and the presence of large numbers of white blood cells. It is designed to get rid of foreign matter, or debris from bruising and injury, which has lodged in our tissues.

If the unwanted matter can be removed, the cells that produce the cytokines should then die. If they do not die then chronic (long-term) inflammation sets in. The severity of the inflammation depends on the prevalence of the different types of cytokines. It can produce symptoms ranging from long-term water retention and weight-gain, to tissue destruction which manifests as arthritis, emphysema, lupus, kidney disease, Crohn's disease, multiple sclerosis and even Alzheimer's disease. In all these diseases, bleach-like toxins produced by white cells during inflammation end up destroying the body's own tissues such as lungs, nerve sheaths, brain cells and kidney tubules, leaving scar tissue in their wake.

A good example of this is acne (spotty skin). If you get spots that remain inflamed for a long time, the acne scars they leave behind can be quite deep. This damage to your skin is not caused by bacteria but by your own immune system, which has remained for too long in inflammatory mode while it tried to get rid of what was irritating your skin.

Gum disease is another example. Pockets of bacteria living off plaque below your gum-line trigger similar inflammation. (If you touch gums affected in this way, you can feel that they are swollen and tender, and they bleed easily.) If your dentist cannot get rid of the bacteria, the inflammation damages the gum from the inside. Your tooth loosens in its socket and may in time fall out.

VITAMIN D AND CYTOKINES

Since the late 1990s, some amazing new discoveries have been made about vitamin D. When it is in short supply, cytokine-producing cells do not die when they are no longer needed. They just go on producing the cytokines which trigger inflammation. The research that led to this remarkable discovery stemmed from trying to find out why multiple sclerosis – the destruction of nerve sheaths caused by chronic inflammation – rarely seems to occur outside northern latitudes where we get little sun and little vitamin D.

The implications of this research are massive, since studies are revealing that high levels of aggressive cytokines appear to be present in a wide range of chronic degenerative diseases. By ensuring a proper vitamin D intake, we may soon be able to prevent or even cure much of this ill-health in the UK, northern Europe and North America.

It seems likely that most people who live in northern latitudes are at risk of vitamin D deficiency, especially if we are health-conscious and avoid full-cream milk, butter and full-fat cheese. Liver has become unpopular as a food due to health scares about its high vitamin A content. In intensive farming (but not in organic farming), large doses of vitamin A supplements are given to animals as a growth promoter, and these build up in the animal's liver. Many of us, especially the elderly and those in nursing homes, prisons etc., spend a lot of time indoors, and when we go out in the sun we cover ourselves and our children with sunscreen products. At northerly latitudes such as the UK, northern Europe and part of North America, the sun for much of the year does not have enough strength to help us make vitamin D.

Recommended Daily Allowances for vitamin D may be enough to prevent rickets in children, but it seems increasingly likely that what is enough to prevent rickets may not be enough to maintain a normal immune system.

Not all vitamin D supplements provide a readily utilizable form of the vitamin. There really is nothing better than good, old-fashioned cod liver oil. If you don't like the taste (and most people don't!) it can be bought in capsule form. Simply take the dose recommended on the label. I would recommend that you buy a purified brand, since PCBs and other ocean pollutants easily become concentrated in fish liver, and high levels of these have been found in some products.

If you suffer from any kind of food intolerance or inflammatory condition and decide to try taking cod liver oil, I would be glad to know if it brings you any benefits. You can let me know by visiting my internet forum at www.health-diets.net.

HEALTH PROBLEMS LINKED WITH INFLAMMATION

Allergies	Inflammation caused by a specific trigger
Alzheimer's disease	Now considered primarily an inflammatory condition which affects parts of the brain
Asthma	Inflammation of the lungs' bronchial tubes
Coeliac disease	Inflammation causing erosion of the small intestine
Colitis	Chronic inflammation of the large intestine
Crohn's disease	Inflammation causing damage to the lower part of the small intestine
Cystitis	Inflammation of the bladder
Eczema	Inflammation of the skin
Emphysema	Inflammation of the lungs' alveoli (the oxygen absorption surfaces)
Gum disease	Inflammation of the gums
Hepatitis	Inflammation of the liver
Irritable bowel syndrome	Temporary inflammation of the large intestine
Lupus	Disseminated inflammation (skin, joints, organs)
Multiple sclerosis	Inflammation of the nerves

Nephrotic syndrome	Inflammation of the kidneys
Osteoarthritis	Inflammation of the joints
Psoriasis	Inflammation of the skin
Rheumatoid arthritis	Inflammation of the joints
Sinusitis	Inflammation of the sinuses

To help your immune system, try to eat at least one bowl of soup a day containing one or more of the power foods listed in the table below. Good ones to start with are Soup 2: Avocado and banana soup with almonds and strawberries, Soup 8: Rejuvenation soup, and Soup 11: Spicy cabbage soup with cod and garlic.

POWER SOUPS FOR A HEALTHY IMMUNE SYSTEM

Power food	What it does	Soup number
Broccoli, Brussels sprouts and kale	Good sources of vitamin C	8, 33, 35
Cayenne (chilli) pepper	Has antiseptic properties. Warms the circulation and helps get oxygen and nutrients to the tissues. Reports suggest it is especially helpful for AIDS sufferers	11, 15, 17, 30, 37, 39, 45, 47, 49, 57, 59, 60, 61
Chicken meat	Good source of protein and zinc	8, 37, 46, 48, 61
Chicken carcass (boiled)	Good source of glucosamine, which has anti-inflammatory properties. Also good source of protein and minerals	8
Chicken liver	Good source of vitamins A, B$_6$ and D, protein, iron, zinc	8
Citrus fruit and juices	Good sources of vitamin C	2, 8, 15, 16, 29, 45, 47, 48, 49, 51, 52, 58, 60, 61
Fish and seafood	Good source of protein, zinc and selenium	11, 36, 46, 53, 54, 55, 57, 60
Garlic	Use raw to benefit from its antibacterial properties. Especially helpful for AIDS sufferers	8, 9, 11, 12, 14, 28, 39, 43, 45, 47, 49, 50, 51, 55, 56, 57, 60

Power food	What it does	Soup number
Ginger	A Yang tonic with anti-inflammatory properties. Warms the circulation	6, 8, 11, 25, 38, 44, 48, 49, 53, 60
Kiwi fruit	Good source of vitamin C	6. Or use as a garnish for other fruit soups
Red and green sweet peppers	Excellent sources of vitamin C	17, 28, 34, 44
Lemon, lime or orange peel or zest	Good source of flavonoids, which have anti-inflammatory properties	1, 16, 29, 45, 47, 57
Lime juice	Is said to help relieve the aches and pains of influenza	15, 47, 51, 60, 61
Onions	Have antiviral and anti-inflammatory properties	Most of our recipes contain onions
Sage	Has antiseptic and anti-inflammatory properties	25
Shiitake mushrooms	Have significant antiviral properties. Also said to contain vitamin D	39, 41, 44
Turmeric	Has powerful anti-inflammatory properties	8, 30, 45, 48

AMAZING DISCOVERIES ABOUT FOOD AND IMMUNITY

1987 Research Reported in the *Journal of Environmental Research*

Selenium affects all components of the immune system. A deficiency of selenium has been shown to lower resistance to bacterial and viral infections, and impairs the production of antibodies and the reproduction, function and effectiveness of white cells. On the other hand, supplementation with selenium has been shown to stimulate all these functions.

Kiremidjian-Schumacher L. et al. *Environ Res* 1987;42(2):277–303.

1995 Research Reported in the *Journal of Acquired Immune Deficiency Syndrome*

In 95 HIV-positive patients, the lower the levels of selenium found in their blood serum, the higher were their rates of death and opportunistic infection. Their serum selenium levels predicted their prognosis more accurately than even their white blood cell count.

Constans J. et al. *J Acquir Immune Defic Syndr Hum Retrovirol* 1995;10(3):392.

1987 Research Reported in the Journal *Federation Proceedings*

Natural killer (NK) cells, which form part of the body's immune system, are known spontaneously to destroy tumour cells and virus-infected cells, and to play a primary role in surveillance. Volunteers were given daily supplements of either raw or aged garlic. Compared with untreated controls, the NK cell performance increased in both garlic-treated groups, by 139 per cent in the raw garlic group and by 155.5 per cent in the aged garlic group.

Kandi O.M. et al. *Fed Proc* 1987;46(3):441.

1989 Research Reported at the International Conference of AIDS (Canada)

Ten HIV-positive patients with advanced AIDS and with infections such as cryptosporidial diarrhoea were given 5 grams daily for six weeks and then 10 grams daily for six weeks of an aged garlic extract. Three patients died before the trial ended, but seven of the 10 experienced a return to normal natural killer cell activity by the end of the 12 weeks. Chronic diarrhoea and candidiasis also improved.

Abdullah T. et al. *Int Conf AIDS (Canada)* 1989;5:466
(ISBN 0-662-56670-X).

1983 Research Reported in the *International Journal of Vitamin and Nutrition Research*

A review of cancer and vitamin C found that vitamin C given to humans in high doses stimulates the immune system in the following ways: by augmenting the activity of white blood cells by 100–300 per cent, by stimulating interferon production, and by significantly raising the serum levels of IgA, IgM and C-3 complement.

Hanck A.: Vitamin C and cancer. *Int J Vit Nutr Res*, Suppl 24: Vitamins in Medicine: Recent Therapeutic Aspects. A Hanck (Ed), pp 87–104, 1983.

1992 Research from the Memorial University of Newfoundland, Canada

Supplementation with a modest amount of vitamins and minerals improved several immune factors and decreased the risk of infection in a controlled trial on elderly people. The treated group had less than half the risk of infection compared with the untreated placebo group.

Chandra R.K. *Lancet* 340:1124–27, 1992.

1993 Research from the Nutritional Immunology Laboratory, USDA Human Nutrition Research Center on Aging, Tufts University, Boston, USA

Animal and human studies suggest that vitamin B6 deficiency impairs immune responses, including the production of antibodies and the reproduction and development of white cells. Vitamin B6 deficiency has been found in elderly people with reduced immunity, HIV-positive individuals, and those with rheumatoid arthritis.

Rall L.C. et al. *Nutr Rev* 1993;51(8):217–25.

1988 Research Reported in the *Journal of the American Medical Association*

Low zinc status has been demonstrated in AIDS sufferers and may cause failure to produce thymic hormone, which plays an important role in immunity.

Fabris N. et al. *JAMA* 1988;259(6):839–840.

SOUP FOR A HEALTHY
CIRCULATION

Most of us think of our circulation as just something which governs how warm or cold we feel. In fact, your circulation involves just about every possible aspect of your health. If the blood supply to your feet and hands is a bit sluggish, you just feel cold. But if part of it shuts off entirely, you could lose a toe or finger.

The same applies to other parts of your body. If the blood supply to the delicate mechanisms of your ears becomes obstructed, deafness will develop. If the blood supply to the memory centre of your brain gets restricted, memory loss and Alzheimer's disease develop. If the blood supply to your heart muscle shuts down, you experience a heart attack. Virtually no part of your body is able to function properly without an adequate supply of blood. Blood carries oxygen and nutrients through arteries and then along thousands of tiny capillary networks, which deliver this precious cargo to each individual cell in your tissues. Whether the cells belong to your liver, heart, kidneys, muscles, nerves, brain or eyes, they cannot survive without oxygen. If a few cells die, you will not notice, as they can be replaced. But if the oxygen starvation continues, more and more cells will die and eventually you will notice a malfunction.

WHAT DAMAGES THE CIRCULATION?

Most of us know that cholesterol deposits can develop on the walls of the coronary arteries that supply the heart. If these deposits become too thick, the blood flow is restricted, and the heart muscle cells get starved of oxygen. You may feel okay while you are resting, but when you try to walk upstairs, the oxygen starvation becomes critical, and you develop a pain in your chest. This pain is known as angina. If your coronary arteries get even more clogged, you may feel chest pain after walking only a few steps.

The medical treatment for this condition is to administer drugs which help to relax your arteries and slow your heart rate. These drugs can make you feel cold and depressed. In men they are prone to cause impotence. People often assume that such drugs are a cure for their condition. If you ask your doctor, he or she will confirm that they are not. They are prescribed to help you cope with your health condition, not to cure it. (Despite this, for safety reasons you should never stop taking a prescribed medicine without your doctor's permission.)

If you are young and strong enough, you may eventually be offered a bypass operation. This creates a new blood supply to your heart, which bypasses the blockages. Again, it is a temporary solution, as the new arteries often become clogged up in a few years. Likewise angioplasty, a procedure that involves scraping out the blocked arteries, does not normally have a lasting effect.

CHOLESTEROL

Many doctors need to update the nutrition advice they give their patients. Amazingly, the old idea that 'if you eat cholesterol it will stick to your arteries and cause heart attacks' is still widely prevalent. Men and women everywhere are trying to follow low-cholesterol diets, cutting out eggs, liver and shellfish, and even worrying that the tiny traces of cholesterol in some cooking oils may give them a heart attack.

Modern nutritionists are trying to get the message across that eating an occasional egg or a piece of liver is not the problem. The cholesterol that does the damage is actually made within your own liver. The four main dietary factors that encourage high cholesterol levels in your body are:

- An excess of foods rich in saturated fat
- An excess of sugary foods and drinks
- A lack of fibre-rich foods
- A lack of leafy green vegetables

SATURATED FATS AND TRANS FATS

Eating too much of the saturated fat found in meat and dairy products is likely to raise cholesterol and make your blood sticky and prone to forming clots. Trans fats, formed in commercial products when fats are processed and hydrogenated, are also linked with raised blood cholesterol levels. Most saturated fat in your diet is not the fat you can see. Foods such as cakes, biscuits, cookies, brownies, pastries, pie-crusts, deep-fried foods, burgers, sausages, cheese, chocolate, ice-cream, creamy sauces, dips and desserts contain enormous amounts of hidden fat – easily 50–70 per cent of their total calorie content. Hidden fat is the real problem. If you've got that under control, it will do you no harm to spread a bit of butter on your toast for breakfast.

SUGARY FOODS AND DRINKS

I have already mentioned on page 7 that consuming sugar raises your insulin levels. The reason why high insulin encourages you to gain weight is that it raises levels of fats in your blood. It also leads to higher cholesterol levels and water retention which raises blood pressure. If you cut down on fat but still consume sugary foods or soft drinks, and sugary tea or coffee several times a day, your cholesterol and blood pressure could still remain high.

DIETARY FIBRE

This helps to keep your bowel motions regular. If you don't have daily bowel motions, then bile salts, which are released by your gall bladder into your intestines to aid digestion, may be reabsorbed from your intestines into your blood and returned to your liver to be converted to cholesterol. If, on the other hand, you eat a diet rich in fibre – especially the soluble fibre found in oats and beans – bile salts will be excreted in your stools, and this helps to prevent cholesterol levels from rising too high.

LEAFY GREEN VEGETABLES

These are the best source of an important B-vitamin known as folic acid. Many individuals are now known to have a faulty gene which creates an abnormally high need for folic acid. If this need is not satisfied then a substance called homocysteine is not broken down as it should be. When this happens, blood cholesterol rises to seriously high levels.

I have known people try desperately to cut every trace of fat out of their diet. A low-fat diet is beneficial, but a totally fat-free diet is actually quite harmful, as we all need sufficient fat in the form of essential polyunsaturated oils in our daily diet. Anyone who eats a low-fat, low-sugar, vegetable-rich diet and still has high cholesterol should assume that it is not fat but homocysteine which is the problem. To bring down homocysteine you need to eat large amounts of foods containing folic acid and its co-factors, vitamins B_6 and B_{12}. To be on the safe side, it is also sensible to take a daily B-complex supplement.

Most people with high cholesterol are not yet routinely tested for homocysteine, so you may have to put pressure on your doctor to get this test. If, despite eating plenty of fruit and vegetables, your homocysteine levels are still high, you may actually need a supplement of folic acid and other B-vitamins.

HIGH BLOOD PRESSURE

Another type of circulatory problem is high blood pressure. This occurs when:

- The artery walls are too rigid, due to too much saturated fat and a lack of essential polyunsaturated oils
- The arteries are too narrow, due to heavy cholesterol deposits
- The blood volume is too great, due to water retention from eating too much salt and/or sugar
- The blood is too sticky, due to smoking or consuming too much saturated fat

High blood pressure puts a strain on your heart and kidneys, and puts you at risk of a stroke. Again, although you must not stop taking them without your doctor's permission, the medical drugs prescribed for it are not a cure, and usually have damaging side-effects such as depression or heavy losses of minerals from your body.

HEART SPASMS

Not all heart attacks are caused by clogged arteries. Some years ago, there was a story in the press about a young man of 25 who had a heart attack and died. It turned out that he loved milk and drank at least 3 litres/5 pints every day, having been told that it was good for him. I also personally know two people – one man aged 22 and another in his 50s – who were rushed to hospital with all the symptoms of a heart attack, but were later told that their arteries were fine and they had probably just had a 'panic attack' due to stress. Yet the people in question had not been under any stress.

If you know where to look in the medical literature, you will find reference to 'cardiac spasms', which can be fatal. They are like getting a stitching pain in your chest so severe that you cannot move or breathe. These spasms shut off the blood supply to your heart just like a heart attack, but are brought on by an imbalance between calcium and magnesium. Most people eat a very magnesium-poor diet. If at the same time you over-consume dairy products, which are very rich in calcium but poor in magnesium, you can aggravate the effects of your magnesium deficiency. The result? Spasms or twitches, irritable nerves and an irregular heartbeat. I have had mild heart spasms myself, in the days before I studied nutrition, when I used to suffer from a magnesium deficiency. They seem to be common. I would bet money on the fact that Prime Minister Tony Blair's 'mysterious' heart condition in 2004 was due to a magnesium deficiency. Magnesium is rapidly depleted by stress, and that was a particularly stressful year for Blair. Why doctors are not taught these things about nutrition we can only guess.

You can avoid getting heart spasms by eating magnesium-rich food every day: fresh vegetables (especially leafy greens), nuts, sunflower seeds, porridge oats, wholemeal bread.

THE MICROCIRCULATION

So far we have mostly discussed problems affecting the arteries. The arteries themselves have only one function: to supply blood to the microcirculation, the capillaries that take oxygen and nutrients directly to the cells themselves.

Your capillary network extends to almost every tissue of your body. Each capillary is about 1 millimetre long, and none of the cells in your body should be more than 0.1 mm away from a capillary. Capillaries are so tiny they can hardly be seen with the naked eye. The capillary itself is a tube whose walls are made up of cells. These cells fit together with narrow gaps or 'pores' between them. On the other side of the capillary wall is the tissue fluid, the watery fluid in your tissue spaces which bathes each of your cells.

Fluid from the capillary is sent out through the pores to join the tissue fluid. Oxygen and nutrients dissolved in this fluid bathe the nearby cells, which absorb what they need. They also release their waste products into the tissue fluid. The used fluid is reabsorbed by the capillaries. Any excess is siphoned off by your lymphatic system, which eventually drains into your veins.

If an artery that supplies blood to one of your capillary networks starts to clog up, the cells can starve. Depending on where the capillaries are, any part of your body – muscles, eyes, ears and so on – could suffer. Some people get pains in their legs if the circulation there becomes restricted. Men with high cholesterol can develop erectile dysfunction (impotence).

A restricted blood flow in your brain can cause a stroke, or a more gradual, progressive loss of brain function. Some researchers are beginning to measure homocysteine levels in people with Alzheimer's disease, and finding them to be high. This means that people suffering from senility may have had circulatory problems for years due to high cholesterol, which was probably not diagnosed if their coronary arteries were not noticeably affected.

LEAKY CAPILLARIES

Problems with your microcirculation can also develop if the walls of your capillaries weaken and their pores widen and become leaky. This happens when your diet is deficient in fruit and vegetables. Flavonoids in these foods are essential for the good health of your capillaries.

Without sufficient flavonoids, your capillaries leak too much fluid into your tissue spaces, and the used fluid cannot get back into the capillaries. The lymphatic system tries to carry it away, but soon becomes overloaded. The result is water retention in your tissues, plus a very sluggish blood supply. Varicose veins are a common symptom. Women can get very heavy menstrual periods due to a flavonoid deficiency. The capillaries in their womb which are meant to release blood actually leak too much blood.

But the microcirculation in the brain, eyes and ears suffers most of all from a lack of flavonoids. This is why dietary supplements made from bilberry extract and ginkgo biloba have been used so successfully in dozens of research studies seeking to improve blood supply in the brain of elderly people. The effectiveness of these supplements against eyesight problems and senility is due to their extremely high content of flavonoids.

To help your heart and circulation, try to eat at least one bowl of soup a day containing one or more of the power foods listed in the table below. Good ones to start with are Soup 3: Baked fruit, cashew and cinnamon soup, Soup 45: Lemon dal soup, and Soup 53: Salmon and potato chunky chowder.

POWER SOUPS FOR A HEALTHY CIRCULATION

Power food	What it does	Soup number
Almonds	Good source of arginine, magnesium, vitamin E and monounsaturated oils (similar to olive oil)	1, 2, 14
Avocado pears	Good source of vitamin B_6, vitamin E and monounsaturated oils	2, 15
Beans and lentils	Rich in B vitamins and soluble fibre	7, 9, 25, 30, 34, 35, 40, 43, 45, 47, 49, 52, 58
Dark red, blue and purple fruits (bilberries, blueberries, blackberries, black cherries, black grapes etc.)	Excellent source of flavonoids	3, 4
Brazil nuts	Good source of selenium	2
Cayenne (chilli) pepper	Good circulatory stimulant	11, 15, 17, 30, 37, 39, 45, 47, 49, 57, 59, 60, 61
Citrus fruit	Good source of vitamin C and flavonoids	2, 8, 15, 16, 29, 45, 47, 48, 49, 51, 52, 58, 60, 61

Power food	What it does	Soup number
Citrus peel or zest	Good source of flavonoids	1, 16, 29, 45, 47, 57
Flax oil	Good source of essential polyunsaturated oils	7, 25 or add one tablespoon to any soup
Garlic	Has cholesterol-lowering properties	8, 9, 11, 12, 14, 28, 39, 43, 45, 47, 49, 50, 51, 55, 56, 57, 60
Ginger	Good circulatory stimulant	6, 8, 11, 25, 38, 44, 48, 49, 53, 60
Leafy greens	Excellent source of folic acid and magnesium	7, 8, 9, 10, 11, 12, 13, 19, 23, 32, 44, 58, 60, 61
Liver	Good source of folic acid and vitamin B_{12}	8
Nuts, sunflower seeds, sesame seeds	Rich in arginine, magnesium, vitamin E, monounsaturated oils and essential polyunsaturated oils	1, 2, 3, 5, 7, 14, 49, 51
Olive oil	Rich in monounsaturated fatty acids	Most of our recipes include olive oil

Power food	What it does	Soup number
Oily fish	For example, salmon, sardines, herrings. Rich in oils that help prevent blood clots.	36, 54. A portion of oily fish can also be eaten with any soup.
Orange juice (freshly squeezed)	Good source of vitamin C and folic acid	Use orange juice in any of the fruit soups
Peanuts	Good source of arginine, which helps to create nitric oxide. This relaxes blood vessels and aids blood flow	46, 59
Pineapple juice	Contains enzymes that help to break down cholesterol deposits in arteries	Use pineapple juice in any of the fruit soups
Soy foods: soy milk, tofu, soy flour, soy sauce, miso	These have significant cholesterol-lowering properties	12, 33, 36, 39, 41, 44, 47, 51

THE BIG HEALTHY SOUP DIET

AMAZING DISCOVERIES ABOUT FOOD AND CIRCULATION

2004 Research from the USDA Human Nutrition Research Center on Aging, Boston, USA

Until quite recently the prevention of coronary heart disease (CHD) has been mostly focused on reducing fat in the diet. Low-fat products are not always helpful, as manufacturers can instead substitute refined carbohydrates. Components in fruit and vegetables, whole grains and nuts help to protect against CHD. Evidence is accumulating that folic acid, vitamin B6, vitamin B12, vitamin E, vitamin C, flavonoids and phyto-oestrogens in particular are highly protective. Olive oil and fish oil are also beneficial. New recommendations, focused on consuming a variety of minimally processed foods, should be developed to prevent heart disease.

Tucker K.L. *Curr Treat Options Cardiovasc Med.* 2004 Aug;6(4):291–302.

2004 Research from the Boston University School of Medicine, USA

The researchers collected data from 4,466 subjects in the National Heart, Lung, and Blood Institute Family Heart Study. The subjects' intake of fruit and vegetables was calculated and compared with their LDL (bad cholesterol) levels. The researchers found that the higher their consumption of fruit and vegetables, the lower their levels of bad cholesterol.

Djousse L. and colleagues. *Am J Clin Nutr.* 2004 Feb;79(2):213–7.

2003 Article from the Kaiser Permanente Center for Health Research, Portland, Oregon, USA

High blood pressure is one of the most important and common risk factors for heart disease and other chronic diseases. Guidelines in the United States recommend that all individuals with high blood pressure should adopt healthy lifestyle habits, including the Dietary Approaches to Stop Hypertension (DASH) diet, to manage their blood pressure. The DASH diet – which is high in fruit, vegetables and low-fat dairy products, and low in fat – has been shown in large trials to reduce blood pressure significantly. The DASH diet has also been shown to reduce blood cholesterol and homocysteine levels.

Craddick S.R. and colleagues. *Curr Atheroscler Rep.* 2003 Nov;5(6):484–91.

2003 Research from the Clinical Nutrition and Risk Factor Modification Center, St Michael's Hospital, Toronto, Canada

LDL (bad) cholesterol can be reduced by consuming almonds regularly, or by eating a diet that is either low in saturated fat or high in soluble fibre, soy protein or plant sterols. The researchers combined all these approaches in a single diet ('portfolio' diet) in order to compare their results with those of recent trials using anti-cholesterol statin drugs. Twenty-five individuals with high LDL levels consumed either the portfolio diet, or a low-fat diet based on whole-wheat cereals and low-fat dairy foods. LDL cholesterol was reduced by 35 per cent on the portfolio diet, but by only 12 per cent on the low-fat diet. The researchers concluded that the portfolio diet was as effective as statin drugs in reducing cholesterol.

Jenkins D.J. and colleagues. *Metabolism.* 2003 Nov;52(11):1478–83.

2004 Research from the Division of Human Nutrition & Epidemiology, Wageningen University, The Netherlands

Mediterranean diets have olive oil as their main source of fat and consist of fruit and vegetables, cereal products, fish, beans and lentils in combination with a little meat and wine with meals. They are low in saturated fat and high in monounsaturated fatty acids, antioxidants (especially vitamins C and E) and high in fibre and folic acid. Mediterranean people enjoy good health and very low mortality rates for coronary heart disease, cancer and other causes. The diet from the Greek island of Crete was tested on heart patients and produced a 70 per cent lower rate of death from heart attack and other causes compared with the standard diet.

Kok F.J. and colleagues. *Eur J Nutr*. 2004 Mar;43 Suppl 1:I/2-5.

1996 Article from the Boston University School of Medicine, USA

Vitamin C can decrease total serum cholesterol levels, increase HDL (good) cholesterol levels, and reduce high blood pressure. Numerous studies have also shown that vitamin C strongly inhibits the oxidation of LDL (bad) cholesterol, which may help to prevent the damage which leads to clogged arteries (atherosclerosis).

Lynch S.M. and colleagues. *Subcell Biochem*. 1996;25:331–67.

1995 Article from the *Journal of the American Medical Association*

Compared with people who consume low amounts of omega-3 polyunsaturated fatty acids from fish and seafood, those consuming at least one meal of oily fish per week have a 50 per cent lower risk of heart attack.

Siscovick D.S. et al. 'Dietary intake and cell membrane levels of long-chain n-3 polyunsaturated fatty acids and the risk of primary cardiac arrest.' *JAMA* 1995;274(17):1363–7.

1995 Article from the *Canadian Journal of Cardiology*

In view of the increasing use of drug therapy in heart disease, advice merely to reduce saturated fat and increase exercise is now thought inadequate. An increased consumption of leafy green vegetables, nuts, seeds and pulses is required to take into account the beneficial effects of soluble fibre, vegetable protein, antioxidants, flavonoids, extra amounts of alpha-linolenic acid, and monounsaturated fats, all of which fight the causes of heart disease.

Jenkins D.J. Optimal diet for reducing the risk of arteriosclerosis. *Can J Cardiol* 1995;11 Suppl G:118G–122G.

1991 Article from the *Journal of Nutritional Medicine*

In 100 patients with high blood pressure treated with a meat-free diet of unrefined grains, fruit, vegetables, nuts, oils and cottage cheese, the average systolic and diastolic blood pressures dropped significantly by 10 mmHg after eight weeks.

Singh R.B. et al. Can dietary changes modulate blood pressure and blood lipids in hypertension? *J Nutr Med* 1991;2:17–24.

1987 Article from the *American Journal of Clinical Nutrition*

The diets of 615 men were investigated and compared with blood pressure readings. A low intake of magnesium was most strongly correlated with higher blood pressure. The authors conclude that vegetables, fruits, whole grains and low-fat dairy items offer protection against high blood pressure.

Am J Clin Nutr 1987;45(2):469–75.

2004 Research from the University Department of Neurology, Ulm, Germany

Dementia rates rise rapidly after the age of 65, and this will become a great burden if nothing is done. Prevention is neglected and treatment has little effect. Contrary to widespread opinion, prevention is possible. Genetic factors account for only about 3 per cent of cases. The importance of the blood circulation is underestimated because impaired microcirculation in the brain is mostly not perceived by the patient. All the risk factors for Alzheimer's disease after the age of 65 are also risk factors for the circulation and especially the microcirculation: Apo-E4, reduced oestrogen, insulin resistance, diabetes, high blood pressure, high cholesterol, old age and increased plasma homocysteine. A healthy lifestyle with daily outdoor activity and a Mediterranean diet not only reduces the risk of dementia, but also of heart attack and cancer.

Kornhuber H.H. *Gesundheitswesen.* 2004 May;66(5):346–51.

SOUP FOR HEALTHY
BONES & JOINTS

HEALTH OF BONES

If asked what type of nourishment is needed for bones, most people would probably still give the same answer as they have for the last 50 years: 'calcium and vitamin D'. Despite the fact that scientists have recently found out a lot more about the nutritional needs of bones, there is sadly an ongoing epidemic of osteoporosis (the bone-thinning disease) in Western society.

Good nutrition is important for joints too, and with the knowledge we have today there is really no valid reason why arthritis should still be affecting 90 per cent of people over the age of 70.

One of the most important functions of bone is to store calcium so that it is readily available for your nervous system, which is extremely sensitive to calcium shortages. In fact, without sufficient calcium, you would develop convulsions. If levels of calcium in your blood drop too low for the health of your nervous system, your parathyroid glands (which are located in your throat behind your thyroid gland) tell your bones to release some calcium into your blood. Once you have had a meal containing sufficient calcium, your bones will get their calcium back. But if the calcium shortage continues, calcium just goes on and on being 'borrowed'. Blood tests show normal calcium readings, but your bones become demineralized, leading eventually to osteoporosis.

This is why calcium is so important for bone health. But modern research (see page 103) is revealing that you cannot prevent or treat osteoporosis just by drinking a lot of milk or taking calcium supplements. That's because a whole host of other nutrients is also important.

Vitamin D

You have probably heard that vitamin D (one of the main vitamins in cod liver oil) is important for bones and is needed to prevent rickets – a softness of the bones that causes deformities in children and used to be widespread in poor communities in northern Europe. Why northern Europe? Vitamin D is also the 'sunshine vitamin'. If you get enough sunlight on your skin, your body can make its own vitamin D.

Without sufficient vitamin D, bones soften and develop osteoporosis because this nutrient is needed for the absorption of all minerals (not just calcium) from your digestive system. Bones lacking in minerals break easily and ache constantly. Children with a vitamin D deficiency develop knock-knees, bow-legs, and a deformed ribcage and skull.

If you live in a northern climate, rarely go outdoors, and don't take cod liver oil, what are your chances of getting enough vitamin D to prevent osteoporosis? Forty years ago drinking a lot of milk might have helped, because only full-fat milk was available to buy, and dairy fat does contain a little vitamin D. But nowadays we mostly buy skimmed or low-fat milk. So-called oily fish (such as herrings, sardines and mackerel) are a good source of vitamin D, but most people do not eat them regularly, if at all.

Vitamin K

Let's assume you are getting plenty of calcium and vitamin D. Do your bones have a healthy old age to look forward to? Not necessarily. Vitamin K has come to the forefront of bone research in recent years. It used to be assumed that bacteria in our intestines could make all the vitamin K we need. Now it seems this is not exactly true as this vitamin K is not absorbable.

If calcium makes for the strength of bones, and vitamin D is needed to absorb calcium from your food, vitamin K is the 'magnet' or 'glue' that helps calcium to stick in place. Without sufficient vitamin K, calcium will just float around, and your bones will not be able to use it. So vitamin K deficiency can also be a major cause of osteoporosis.

The best sources of vitamin K are cauliflower, Brussels sprouts, cabbage and other leafy greens. You can get small amounts from a variety of different foods, but if my bones were at stake I would not leave this to chance. It is so easy to make delicious soups with the very best sources of vitamin K, so why take any risks?

Collagen-forming Nutrients

You have probably heard of collagen in connection with your skin. Bones contain collagen too. It is a type of protein, and in bones it is the foundation to which calcium clings. Amino acids, vitamin C, zinc, copper, manganese and silicon are all needed to form bone collagen. Flavonoids from dark blue and purple berries are noted for their beneficial effects on stabilizing collagen.

Again, you risk developing osteoporosis if any of these nutrients are lacking in your diet. Without collagen, there is nothing for calcium to cling to.

The Menopause

Since women mainly seem to get osteoporosis after the menopause, it has become customary for doctors to prescribe artificial hormones (HRT) for this condition. They assume that their patients are already doing their best to eat the right diet, in line with official recommendations and with the advice given by dieticians and nursing staff. Because their doctor has prescribed it, most women seem to feel safe taking HRT despite the known cancer risks. The longer you take HRT, the more the risk rises; and when you stop taking it, osteoporosis can quickly set in if your diet has been faulty.

Until doctors stop treating HRT as a safe and effective alternative to proper nutritional advice, women will continue getting osteoporosis and society will carry on paying massive costs for the care of elderly people with broken hip-bones. As you can see from the research studies on page 103, osteoporosis is not a low-oestrogen problem. Many of the health problems that mainly occur after the menopause, such as breast cancer and fibroids, are problems caused by too *much* oestrogen rather than too little. Oestrogen is made not just by your ovaries, but by your adrenal glands and body fat too. Even men make some oestrogen.

As long as conventional medical treatments are based on faulty, over-simplified concepts, I would recommend questioning everything you are told, and always getting second opinions from doctors who specialize in natural medicine (see Resources, page 277).

On the other hand, plant foods rich in phyto-oestrogens have proven benefits for women after the menopause. The best ones are soy foods, rice, sage leaf and virgin olive oil.

Other Causes of Bone Loss

Lack of exercise
It is well known that a lack of exercise encourages osteoporosis. Regular running, fast walking, swimming, aerobics, dancing or gym work can not only help to prevent it, but research has shown that bones can even gain density if you exercise more.

Smoking
Smoking depletes the body of antioxidants and has multiple harmful effects on health. Research has shown that smoking also causes osteoporosis, especially in hip-bones.

Eating too much protein
Habitually eating more than about 4 ounces (100 grams) of protein with each meal makes your blood acidic. Extra calcium has to be mobilized from your bones to neutralize this acidity; this calcium is then lost in your urine. (This is one of the risks of following low-carbohydrate diets on a long-term basis.)

Consuming too many sugary foods and drinks
These cause increased losses of calcium through your urine. The reason for this is not clear.

Consuming too many soft drinks

Large amounts of phosphorus are found in most carbonated drinks and effervescent tablets. Extra calcium has to be mobilized from your bones to neutralize this phosphorus; this calcium is then lost in your urine.

Excess salt and coffee

Both these items speed up your excretion of minerals through your urine, and research shows a link with osteoporosis.

High homocysteine levels in the blood

You may remember from page 82 that homocysteine is a harmful substance encouraged by B-vitamin deficiencies, and leads to high cholesterol levels. It can also play a part in the development of osteoporosis.

HEALTH OF JOINTS

As you probably know, your joints are areas where bones are held together with ligaments and cartilage. The function of cartilage is to protect joints, and most long-term health problems involving the joints are caused by the loss of cartilage.

You may be surprised to learn that cartilage is mostly water. The water is held in a slippery, highly absorbent complex consisting of glucosamine and cartilage-producing cells. The water content is high because water is good at absorbing impact and so helps to protect the joint.

Cartilage loss occurs when joints become irritated and inflammation sets in (see the section on the immune system for more about this). Causes of irritation include excess pressure and friction, combined with cartilage shrinking due to dehydration. A common problem in Western society, dehydration often goes unnoticed. It occurs from drinking too little plain water, and too much tea, coffee and alcohol, all of which are diuretics, and make you continue excreting water even when you are already getting dehydrated.

As cartilage is worn away, eventually bone rubs on bone, which maintains a long-term irritation. Painful little bony spurs can develop on the unprotected joint surface. This condition is known as osteoarthritis.

Food intolerances are a major cause of chronic inflammation in joints. Many people are intolerant to wheat or dairy products. Some arthritis sufferers are made worse by acidic foods and citrus fruit, others by foods in the deadly nightshade family: potatoes, peppers and tomatoes. Eating too many salty foods encourages irritation as a result of higher histamine levels.

There are other types of arthritis, including rheumatoid arthritis, which involves the presence of aggressive cytokines (see page 70) which target the joints.

Medical treatments consist mostly of painkillers and anti-inflammatory drugs. They are not a cure, and they all have side-effects. On the other hand, natural treatments have brought cures for thousands of people. The best results come from working with a reputable practitioner, but if you have arthritis, there are plenty of soup ingredients that will help to combat this problem. I would especially recommend that you experiment with eating just the soups marked as compatible with the Waterfall Diet (see page 131). Many cases diagnosed as arthritis are just painful water retention around the joints, and this diet is specifically designed to release water retention.

To help combat bone and joint problems, try to eat at least one bowl of soup a day containing one or more of the foods listed in the table on pages 101–102. Good ones to start with are Soup 7: Potage of celery and parsley, Soup 8: Rejuvenation soup, and Soup 33: Broccoli cream soup with Stilton cheese.

POWER SOUPS FOR HEALTHY BONES AND JOINTS

Power food	What it does	Soup number
Cabbage, broccoli, Brussels sprouts and other green vegetables	Rich in calcium and vitamin K. Also rich in folic acid, which helps combat homocysteine	7, 8, 9, 10, 11, 12, 13, 19, 23, 32, 33, 35, 40, 44, 58, 60, 61
Celery	Helps to reduce water retention and inflammation	7, 23, 43, 55, 57
Chicken carcass (boiled)	Natural source of glucosamine, which attracts water into cartilage and stimulates cells to begin rebuilding cartilage	8
Chicken liver	Rich in folic acid, vitamin B$_{12}$, iron and zinc	8
Cider vinegar	Traditional anti-arthritis remedy	14, 39. Can also be added to other soups
Dairy products (milk, cheese, yoghurt)	Rich in calcium. Butter and cream also contain a little vitamin D	1, 2, 4, 5, 6, 12, 15, 19, 28, 33, 34, 54, 56
Dark red, blue and purple fruits (bilberries, blueberries, blackberries, black cherries, black grapes etc.)	Rich in vitamin C. Also have anti-inflammatory properties	3, 4

Power food	What it does	Soup number
Gelatine	Provides raw materials to help rebuild cartilage	8 (from boiling bones and cartilage). Commercial gelatine can be added to any soup
Ginger	Has anti-inflammatory properties	6, 8, 11, 25, 38, 44, 48, 49, 53, 60
Nuts, sunflower seeds, sesame seeds	Rich in calcium, magnesium and zinc	1, 2, 3, 5, 7, 14, 49, 51
'Oily' fish (salmon, sardines, herrings etc.)	Good source of vitamin D	36, 54. A portion of oily fish can also be eaten with any soup
Onions	Rich in quercetin, which has anti-inflammatory properties	Most of our recipes contain onion
Turmeric (yellow Indian spice)	Research shows that its anti-inflammatory properties may be as strong as those of the drug phenylbutazone	8, 30, 45, 48

AVOID DEHYDRATION

The health of your joints starts with drinking WATER. Drink eight glasses (2 litres) a day. The water should be drunk plain so that it has the capacity to absorb the wastes dissolved in your blood.

AMAZING DISCOVERIES ABOUT
FOOD AND BONE HEALTH

2004 Research from the University of Aberdeen, UK

Many women lose bone density rapidly around the time of the menopause. In this research study, 891 women were evaluated at age 45–55 for diet and bone density, and followed up seven years later. The women who consumed more fruit and vegetables and calcium-rich foods lost bone more slowly than the women who consumed the most fat.

Macdonald H.M. and colleagues. *Am J Clin Nutr.* 2004 Jan;79(1):155–65.

2004 Research from the University of Southern California and The Orthopedic Hospital, Los Angeles, USA

Magnesium deficiency increases the risk of developing osteoporosis. According to the US Department of Agriculture, the average daily intake of magnesium suggests that a substantial number of people may be at risk of magnesium deficiency, especially if any aggravating factors and/or medications deplete their magnesium status even further.

Rude R.K. and colleagues. *J Nutr Biochem.* 2004 Dec;15(12):710–6.

1991 Article from the *Journal of Nutritional Medicine*

The effect of magnesium-emphasized supplementation on bone density in a group of post-menopausal women using hormone-replacement therapy was 16 times greater than that of dietary advice alone.

Abraham G.E. *J Nutr Med* 1991;2:165–178.

1988 Research from the Garvan Institute of Medical Research, Sydney, Australia

The intake of 14 nutrients was measured in 159 women aged 23–75 and compared with bone mineral density. A high calcium intake did not appear to be particularly protective. The best levels of bone density were found in individuals with the highest intakes of magnesium, zinc and iron.

Angus R.M. and colleagues. *Bone Miner* 1988;4(3):265–77.

1994 Research from the Department of Biology, University of California at San Diego, USA

Fifty-nine healthy post-menopausal women were given daily supplements of (1) calcium, (2) calcium plus zinc, manganese and copper, or (3) dummy pills (placebo). Their bones were monitored for two years while they took these supplements. The researchers found that, compared with the placebo, the calcium supplements on their own showed no benefits. But the combined calcium plus trace minerals group showed a significantly slower rate of bone loss than the placebo group.

Strause L. and colleagues. *J Nutr* 1994;124(7):1060–4.

1993 Research from the Hôpital Edouard Herriot, Lyon, France

Blood vitamin K levels were found to be much lower in 51 elderly women with hip fractures compared to those with healthy bones. Many of them had undetectable levels of vitamin K. The investigators conclude that vitamin K deficiency puts elderly patients at risk of hip fracture.

Hodges S.J. and colleagues. *J Bone Miner Res* 8(10):1241–5, 1993.

2003 Research from the Department of Sports Medicine, School of Medicine, Keio University, Tokyo, Japan

It is established in Japan that treatment with vitamin D_3 (the form of vitamin D found in cod liver oil) helps to maintain bone density and prevent fractures in the spinal bones of post-menopausal women with osteoporosis. Vitamin K supports many functions in the body which help bone to regenerate. It has been shown to help maintain the density of bones in the lower back, and to prevent bone fractures in patients with osteoporosis. Its effects are reduced when levels of vitamin D_3 are inadequate. This is why treatments using each vitamin separately have not always been successful. These researchers believe that if both vitamins are prescribed together they can reverse age-related bone deterioration.

Iwamoto J. and colleagues. *Keio J Med.* 2003 Sep;52(3):147–50.

2001 Research from the University of Memphis Center for Community Health, Tennessee, USA

In evaluating 86 studies enrolling 40,753 individuals, smokers had a much lower bone density than non-smokers. At the hip in particular, the bone density of current smokers was one-third less than that of people who had never smoked.

Ward K.D. and colleagues. *Calcif Tissue Int,* 2001;68:259–270.

1987 Research from the University of Connecticut, Storrs, USA

The urine of 13 individuals consuming a beverage containing 2 grams of added sugar per kilo of their body weight was analysed. It was found that this sugar caused significant losses of calcium in their urine.

Holl M.G. and colleagues. *J Nutr* 117(7):1229–33, 1987.

1988 Research from Andrews University, Berrien Springs, Michigan, USA

Those who followed a lacto-vegetarian diet for at least 20 years had only 18 per cent less bone by age 80 compared with 35 per cent less bone in meat-eaters.

Marsh A.G. and colleagues. *Am J Clin Nutr* 48(3 Suppl):837–41, 1988.

1995 Research from Creighton University, Omaha, Nebraska, USA

An analysis was made of 560 calcium studies carried out on 190 women aged 34–69. The researchers found that for every 6 fluid ounce (177.5 ml) serving of coffee consumed, an extra 40 mg calcium has to be consumed just to maintain calcium balance.

Barger-Lux M.J. and colleagues. *Osteoporos Int* 5(2):97–102, 1995.

1998 Article from the *Journal of Nutritional and Environmental Medicine*

High homocysteine levels in the blood (often due to B-complex deficiency) are a major cause of osteoporosis.

McLaren-Howard J. and colleagues. *Journal of Nutritional and Environmental Medicine* 1998;8:129–138.

SOUP FOR HEALTHY
HORMONES

Some of the most exciting new medical research is looking at how your hormones are profoundly affected by what you eat. Hormones govern our metabolism, water balance, reproductive functions, moods and feelings. They help us make energy and cope with stress. By changing our bodies at puberty, they even drastically affect the way we look.

Hormones are made from protein, with the aid of vitamins and minerals. If your diet is low in some of these nutrients, or if you are not properly absorbing them, then your hormones are at risk. This can result in a whole host of health problems, from chronic fatigue to premenstrual syndrome (PMS), infertility and diabetes.

Soup can boost nourishment for your glands, which produce your hormones. By adding concentrated ingredients like vegetable juices to soup, you can double or treble your vitamin and mineral intake. What a mouth-watering way to take your vitamins!

Now let's take a look at some of the glands and hormones that are linked with everyday health problems, and how nutrition can help them.

ADRENAL HORMONES

Related health issues: fatigue, weakness, depression, coldness, dizziness on standing, allergies, a desire for salty food, frequent infections, difficulty coping with stress, reduced sex drive and (for menopausal women) hot flushes.

Your adrenal glands produce several important hormones: adrenaline, noradrenaline, cortisol, aldosterone and small amounts of the sex hormones. Adrenal hormones are made of cholesterol with the help of choline and the amino acids tyrosine and methionine.

Adrenaline keeps your mind and body alert and your mood high. You make more adrenaline when you are under stress. This prepares your body for physical activity and increases your metabolic rate.

Under stress you also make more cortisol. If your blood sugar and carbohydrate stores get too low, cortisol can help you to make energy from other foods.

Cortisol is also called into action to calm down an overactive immune system, and it can block allergic reactions. If you get a lot of allergic reactions, accompanied by dark circles around and under your eyes, it is possible that your adrenals are underactive – a condition known as hypoadrenia. Overstressed glands can become exhausted when they lack sufficient raw materials from your diet. (See the list of adrenal stressors on page 109.)

Another potential sign of hypoadrenia can be frequent urination. Your adrenals make a hormone called aldosterone to prevent you from urinating too much and getting dehydrated. So if you find yourself constantly drinking and urinating, and if your doctor has ruled out diabetes (which can also cause this problem), you might be producing insufficient aldosterone as a result of hypoadrenia.

Hypoadrenia is closely related to hypothyroidism, and has many similar symptoms, including a tendency to weakness, fatigue and low body temperature. Cells in the thyroid gland are able to interact with adrenaline. Researchers are also beginning to reveal connections between adrenal hormones and female sex hormones, which could help them discover the real cause of menopausal hot flushes.

What Stresses Your Adrenals

- Constant anxiety or other negative emotions
- Sleep deprivation
- Excessive exercise
- Trauma and infections
- Allergic reactions and food intolerances
- Intestinal toxins (e.g. from yeast and bacterial overgrowth)
- Environmental toxins and pollutants (including smoking, and mercury from tooth fillings)
- Occupational toxins
- Overconsumption of sugary foods and drinks
- Caffeine, alcohol and smoking
- Inadequate protein, vitamins and minerals

These stressors increase the nutritional needs of your adrenal glands, and a high-stress, junk-diet lifestyle eventually takes its toll. Consuming too many sugary foods and drinks is particularly stressful. These push up insulin, which forces your adrenals to work overtime as they try to control it. A diet lacking in magnesium also tends to raise levels of adrenal hormones (see the research summaries on page 25).

What Helps Your Adrenals

- Protein, especially the amino acids tyrosine and methionine
- Folic acid (for tyrosine and methionine metabolism)
- Vitamin B12 (for folic acid metabolism)
- Zinc and copper
- Vitamins B5 and C
- Chromium, magnesium, vitamins B1, B2, B3 (to help control insulin)

Cayenne (chilli) peppers help gently to kick-start the adrenals, and can easily be added to soup. Methionine may be particularly low in the diet of vegetarians who rely mainly on beans, lentils and tofu for protein. On the other hand, nuts and sunflower seeds are a good source of methionine and should always be added to a vegetarian diet. Among the starches, rice is the only good source of methionine, and should be eaten as much as possible in preference to bread, pasta and potatoes.

Babies Born with Hypoadrenia

When a woman with hypoadrenia becomes pregnant, she may feel very tired and nauseous in the first few months but can blossom in late pregnancy, when her baby's adrenal glands are developed enough to produce enough adrenal hormones for two. Then, when she gives birth and suddenly loses her extra supply of adrenal hormones, the mother may collapse with severe postnatal depression. Meanwhile, the baby is born with exhausted adrenal glands and a future of allergies and frequent infections. If you are a woman who is thinking of becoming pregnant, now is the time to start looking after your adrenal glands.

To help your adrenal glands, try to eat at least one bowl of soup a day containing one or more of the power foods listed in the table on pages 111–12. Good ones to start with are Soup 36: Butternut bisque with Cajun-style red mullet, and Soup 46: Malaysian laksa.

POWER SOUPS TO HELP YOUR ADRENAL GLANDS

Power food	What it does	Soup number
Brazil nuts	Rich in zinc, copper and methionine	2
Brown rice	Better than other carbohydrate foods as it contains methionine. Also a source of B-vitamins	8, 11, 23, 24, 29, 37, 50
Cayenne (chilli) pepper	Helps gently to kick-start the adrenals	11, 15, 17, 30, 37, 39, 45, 47, 49, 57, 59, 60, 61
Cheese	A good source of zinc and tyrosine	12, 19, 20, 28, 33
Fish and chicken	Good sources of zinc and tyrosine	8, 11, 36, 37, 46, 48, 53, 54, 55, 57, 60, 61
Leafy green vegetables	A good source of vitamin C and folic acid	7, 8, 9, 10, 11, 12, 13, 19, 23, 32, 44, 58, 60, 61
Liver	A good source of zinc, copper, B-vitamins, amino acids and chromium	8
'Oily' fish: sardines, salmon, herrings, mackerel	Help to prevent overproduction of adrenal hormones in stressful situations	36, 54. A portion of oily fish can also be eaten with any soup

Power food	What it does	Soup number
Peanuts	A good source of zinc and tyrosine	46, 59
Sunflower seeds	Rich in zinc, magnesium and methionine	7

THYROID HORMONE

Related health issues: fatigue, weight gain, coldness, hair loss

Thyroxine, the main hormone produced by your thyroid gland, is responsible for governing your metabolism. Low thyroid function (hypothyroidism) tends to slow down metabolism, but not all hypothyroid people are overweight. Like adrenaline, thyroxine is made from the amino acid tyrosine, with the help of the mineral iodine. These are both vital nutrients for the thyroid gland.

Another important nutrient is iron. Due to menstruation, iron deficiency is common in women. In a study carried out at Pennsylvania State University in 1990, 10 women with iron deficiency anaemia were compared to 12 women with normal iron levels. They were found to have lower body temperatures and lower levels of thyroid hormone. After receiving iron supplements for 12 weeks, the women's body temperatures increased and their thyroid hormone levels returned to near normal.

In order to help make and activate thyroxine your thyroid gland also needs:

- Vitamin A
- Vitamin B1
- Zinc
- Selenium
- Copper

Fluoride – a Thyroid Toxin

Beware of giving fluoride supplements to children, or allowing them to swallow toothpaste containing fluoride. Fluoride inactivates iodine and so can affect the thyroid gland. Some have even linked it with thyroid cancer, and many action groups are calling for the banning of artificial water fluoridation.

Some foods have anti-thyroid effects, especially the soy-based meat substitutes TVP (textured vegetable protein) and soy protein isolate. It may be unsafe to consume them on a daily basis. The same goes for raw cabbage and raw peanuts. Other soy products such as soy milk and tofu can be consumed in moderation.

Hypothyroid people lack the ability to convert beta-carotene to vitamin A, so if you suffer from hypothyroidism you will need to eat some liver occasionally or take cod liver oil supplements.

Thyroid and Oestrogen

Many women have health problems such as fibroids and endometriosis caused by an oestrogen imbalance. Excessively high oestrogen makes your body produce a protein that partially inactivates thyroxine. Your thyroid gland then has to step up producing thyroxine in an effort to maintain normal levels. In time, thyroid exhaustion and hypothyroidism can set in.

One potential cause of high oestrogen is an iodine deficiency. Not only does a lack of iodine reduce your ability to produce thyroxine, but it also seems to deplete thyroxine by stimulating a higher rate of oestrogen production. You can raise your iodine by adding a little seaweed (available in health-food stores) to soup. Many Japanese foods, such as powdered miso soup, contain some seaweed. There is also a small amount of iodine and other minerals in sea salt. See the section on women's hormones for more information (page 115).

In his *Encyclopedia of Healing Juices*, medical anthropologist John Heinerman reports that another helpful food for the thyroid is radishes. According to Russian scientists, these contain a substance called raphanin which helps the thyroid to balance its production of hormones.

To help combat thyroid problems, try to eat at least one bowl of soup a day containing one or more of the power foods listed in the table below. Good ones to start with are Soup 8: Rejuvenation soup, and Soup 25: Broad bean soup with apple and radish.

POWER SOUPS TO HELP THE THYROID

Power food	What it does	Soup number
Beans and lentils	A good source of iron	7, 9, 25, 30, 34, 35, 40, 43, 45, 47, 49, 52, 58
Brazil nuts	Rich in zinc, copper, selenium and methionine	2
Cheese	A good source of zinc and tyrosine	12, 19, 20, 28, 33
Fish and seafood	Good source of iodine, zinc, selenium and tyrosine	11, 36, 46, 53, 54, 55, 57, 60
Liver	A good source of iron, zinc, copper, vitamin A, B-vitamins, amino acids and chromium	8
Meat and chicken	Good sources of tyrosine, iron and zinc	8, 37, 46, 48, 61 (chicken)
Radishes and radish juice	A source of raphanin, which balances the thyroid	25, 44, 60, 61
Seaweed (e.g. nori, wakame, laverbread, arame)	An excellent source of iodine	8, 21, 44

WOMEN'S HORMONES

Related health issues: heavy menstruation, PMS, menopausal hot flushes, breast lumps, endometriosis, polycystic ovaries, breast cancer

The two main female hormones, oestrogen and progesterone, are made in the ovaries. Oestrogen levels rise until ovulation, after which the woman must make more progesterone while her liver breaks down the oestrogen. Some oestrogen is also made in the adrenal glands and in the body fat of both men and women. Oestrogen and progesterone regulate sexual development, ovulation, menstruation and pregnancy.

Most of the health problems listed above seem to be linked with high body levels of oestradiol, the most active form of oestrogen. Excesses of this hormone should be broken down by a woman's liver, but eating the wrong kind of diet can reduce the efficiency of her liver enzymes.

Effects of Excess Oestrogen

Oestrogen stimulates the growth of breasts, ovaries and womb lining, so an excess can encourage breast and ovarian cysts, fibroids, endometriosis and breast cancer. Painful, heavy menstrual periods can also be due to high oestrogen levels.

Unless depression is her main symptom, any woman with premenstrual syndrome (PMS) should be assumed to have high oestrogen levels. Premenstrual depression, on the other hand, is more likely to be linked with *low* oestrogen levels. This is because low oestrogen leads to higher levels of enzymes which break down adrenaline. The resulting lack of adrenaline is the cause of the depression. Taking antibiotics can greatly increase oestrogen excretion and so lead to low oestrogen levels.

Reducing High Oestrogen

Foods rich in B-vitamins and the amino acid methionine help your liver to break down excessive oestrogen. Likewise, foods in the cabbage family, including Brussels sprouts and broccoli, are very helpful. On the

WHAT RAISES OESTROGEN LEVELS?

Consuming too much dairy produce	Cow's milk and its products are high in natural oestrogen
Consuming too much grapefruit or grapefruit juice	Blocks liver enzymes which break down oestrogen
Consuming traces of organochlorine pesticides	These act as oestrogen mimics with many times the potency of natural oestrogen
Eating too much fat and meat	Encourages intestinal bacteria which reduce oestrogen excretion
Having too much body fat	Oestrogen is partly produced by body fat
Not eating enough brassica vegetables (cabbage, broccoli, Brussels sprouts, cauliflower)	These vegetables help a woman's liver to break down oestrogen
Not eating enough dietary fibre	Fibre is needed for you to excrete excess oestrogen
Not eating enough foods rich in B-vitamins (oatmeal, wholemeal bread, brown rice, beans)	Liver enzymes need B-vitamins
Not eating enough foods rich in iodine (fish and seafood, seaweed)	Iodine deficiency seems to stimulate higher oestrogen production

other hand, grapefruit and grapefruit juice contain naringenin, which blocks the liver enzymes that metabolize oestrogen.

The weak 'plant oestrogens' in soy foods compete with stronger body oestrogens for absorption. This reduces uptake of the latter, thus reducing total body oestrogen.

High-fibre foods can help to reduce oestrogen by binding to it in the gut and preventing its reabsorption.

Your diet should also be low in fat, and should avoid dairy products, which are the highest source of dietary oestrogen. Fish or seaweed products should be regularly consumed for their iodine content.

The Menopause

It is not widely known that the adrenal glands make testosterone in both men and women. In women, testosterone is converted to oestrogen. In fact, female sex drive depends on testosterone and not on oestrogen, as is commonly thought. Adrenal exhaustion can greatly reduce sex drive in women.

Although we assume that women can no longer make sex hormones after the menopause, when the ovaries stop producing oestrogen, this is not true at all; the adrenal glands continue to produce sex hormones. Although they often occur in later life, problems such as fibroids and breast cancer are actually caused by excessively *high* levels of oestrogen. This means that a lack of oestrogen is unlikely to be the prime cause of menopausal hot flushes, even though taking artificial oestrogen products seems to prevent them.

Since stress tends to bring on hot flushes, scientific researchers are beginning to investigate the possibility that artificial oestrogens help menopausal symptoms only indirectly, perhaps by boosting the effects of cortisol or adrenaline.

The best way to help prevent menopausal problems is to follow the advice given for the adrenal glands.

To help balance oestrogen, try to eat at least one bowl of soup a day containing one or more of the power foods listed in the table on pages 118–19. Good ones to start with are Soup 11: Spicy cabbage soup with cod and garlic, and Soup 44: Japanese buckwheat noodle soup.

POWER SOUPS TO HELP BALANCE OESTROGEN

Power food	What it does	Soup number
Bran cereals	Rich in a type of fibre that aids oestrogen excretion	Bran can be added to most soups
Brown rice	Source of B-vitamins	8, 11, 23, 24, 29, 37, 50
Cabbage family (cabbage, broccoli, Brussels sprouts, cauliflower, watercress)	These help your liver to break down excess oestrogen	8, 9, 10, 11, 12, 13, 32, 33, 35, 40, 44, 61
Fish and seafood	Good source of iodine	11, 36, 46, 53, 54, 55, 57, 60
Liver	A good source of iron, zinc, copper, vitamin A, B-vitamins, amino acids and chromium	8
Oats	Source of B-vitamins	Try adding a teaspoon of oatmeal to some of the bean or vegetable soups
Seaweed (e.g. nori, wakame, laverbread, arame)	An excellent source of iodine	8, 21, 44

Power food	What it does	Soup number
Soy foods: soy milk, tofu, soy flour, soy sauce, miso	Help to prevent your cells from absorbing too much oestrogen	12, 33, 36, 39, 41, 44, 47, 51

INSULIN

I have mentioned the harmful effects of high insulin several times in this book. Insulin is a hormone made by your pancreas. Its job is to carry glucose from your blood into your cells, which can then use the glucose to make energy. This glucose is produced when you digest your food. Most of it comes from carbohydrate foods such as sugar, but even protein and parts of the fat molecule can be turned into glucose if you need it.

In healthy individuals, insulin levels do not stay high unless you keep consuming sugary food or drink many times a day. The sugar in these items gets into your bloodstream very quickly and has to be matched by rapid surges of insulin. As you already know, this insulin can raise your blood fats and cholesterol, and it overworks your adrenal glands (see page 109).

About one third of the population is thought to be particularly 'sugar-sensitive'. These individuals make the most insulin, and are at the highest risk of developing insulin resistance and diabetes (see below).

Insulin Resistance ('Syndrome X')

This is another cause of chronically high insulin levels. It is a pre-diabetic state which only arises in adulthood. Here, insulin seems to go unheeded by your muscle and fat cells. Instead of using the insulin to pick up glucose, your cells ignore it and allow the glucose to remain in your blood. In an attempt to overcome this, your pancreas steps up insulin production, and the result is permanently high insulin levels.

Some of your organs cannot cope with this extra insulin. Too much insulin makes your kidneys retain sodium, causing water retention, high blood pressure and high levels of uric acid. When insulin overstimulates your liver, your blood fats rise, leading to atherosclerosis and heart disease. When there is too much insulin around, a woman's ovaries can begin making more testosterone, leading to symptoms of polycystic ovary syndrome (PCOS). Another effect of high insulin is a change in body shape. Body fat begins to collect mainly in your abdomen and around your waist. At an advanced stage, insulin resistance is known as Type II diabetes. (The other type of diabetes, known as Type I, only affects children, and its cause is unknown.)

WHAT PROMOTES INSULIN RESISTANCE?

Chromium deficiency	Chromium deficiency reduces the ability of insulin to bond to cells. By correcting this deficiency, researchers have been able to improve the uptake of insulin up to threefold
B-complex deficiency	B-vitamins work with chromium to help insulin bond to cells
Magnesium deficiency	Magnesium works alongside B-vitamins
Being overweight	Large amounts of body fat are one of the biggest risk factors for developing insulin resistance
Lack of exercise	Taking exercise – even just walking for half an hour a day – can reduce insulin resistance by up to 40 per cent
High-sugar diet	Consuming sugary foods and drinks produces insulin surges

On pages 122–23 is a list of power foods that can help insulin resistance, but some extra dietary advice is also important. If you suffer from this problem, your diet should consist of small, frequent meals and snacks (whether soup or not) so that your blood sugar stays as even as possible. It is also important not to consume sugary food and drinks, or stimulants such as tea, coffee and alcohol. These make extra demands on insulin and on other hormones involved in blood sugar control. Consuming soups high in soluble fibre, such as found in beans and oatmeal, helps to slow down the absorption of carbohydrates into your blood, as does the presence of a little oil or fat.

If you suffer from insulin resistance, avoid drinking fruit juice unless you dilute it with plenty of water. Fruit itself contains pectin, which slows down absorption of the natural sugars in fruit. But when the fibre is removed to make juice, these sugars are rapidly absorbed unless the juice is consumed with a balanced meal.

To help prevent insulin resistance and diabetes, try to eat at least one bowl of soup a day containing one or more of the power foods listed in the table on pages 122–23. Good ones to start with are Soup 35: Brussels butterbean bisque, and Soup 49: Mung bean soup with garlic and ginger.

POWER SOUPS TO HELP PREVENT INSULIN RESISTANCE AND DIABETES

Power food	What it does	Soup number
Beans and lentils	Rich in B-vitamins and in soluble fibre which helps to slow down the absorption of natural sugars into your blood	7, 9, 25, 30, 34, 35, 40, 43, 45, 47, 49, 52, 58
Cinnamon	Contains methylhydroxy chalcone polymer (MHCP), which has been shown to help glucose metabolism	3, 5, 30
Fenugreek seeds (powdered)	There is some evidence that these can help glucose metabolism	30, 52
Leafy green vegetables	A good source of magnesium	7, 8, 9, 10, 11, 12, 13, 19, 23, 32, 44, 58, 60, 61
Liver	A good source of chromium	8
Oats	Rich in B-vitamins, magnesium, chromium and soluble fibre	Try adding a teaspoon of oatmeal to some of the bean or vegetable soups
'Oily' fish: sardines, salmon, herrings, mackerel	Rich in B-vitamins, zinc and oils which help to protect your arteries and heart from the effects of high insulin	36, 54. A portion of oily fish can also be eaten with any soup.

Power food	What it does	Soup number
Psyllium husks	Rich in soluble fibre	39
Sesame seeds (ground or as tahini paste)	A good source of magnesium, zinc and fibre	49
Sunflower seeds	A good source of magnesium and zinc	7

PROSTATE ENLARGEMENT

This is a problem that can affect men from middle age onwards. Men with an enlarged prostate gland find it difficult to empty their bladder. They may have to get up several times every night to urinate.

Prostate enlargement is usually blamed on increased levels of a male hormone known as DHT, which is related to testosterone. On the other hand, Dr Eugene Shippen, author of the *Testosterone Syndrome,* says that if DHT is administered artificially, the prostate actually shrinks. This means that some other cause of prostate enlargement is more likely. Functional medicine expert Dr Jeffrey Bland suggests that research should be carried out investigating possible links with insulin. Insulin makes a plausible culprit as it stimulates cell growth and the production of male hormones.

What Helps the Prostate?

Enlarged prostate glands can respond very well to a change in diet. Special foods that help the prostate include pumpkin seeds, soy foods and tomatoes.

One of the oils in pumpkin seeds, known as delta-7-sterol, is especially therapeutic as it has been shown to help prevent the prostate cells from absorbing too much DHT. Likewise, soy foods can be as beneficial in balancing male hormones as they are for female hormones.

Pumpkin seeds are also a rich source of zinc and essential fatty acids, which are often deficient in men with prostate enlargement.

A zinc deficiency may be partly to blame for this condition, since zinc supplements – particularly when combined with vitamin B6 and flax oil – have proved to be a successful treatment in many cases. Lycopene, the red pigment in tomatoes, tends to concentrate in the prostate gland. The trace element selenium also appears to be important. There is now research to show that men who eat more tomato products and selenium tend to have lower rates of prostate cancer.

To help combat prostate problems, try to eat at least one bowl of soup a day containing one or more of the power foods listed in the table below. Good ones to start with are Soup 26: Quick and easy cream of tomato soup, and Soup 53: Salmon and potato chunky chowder.

POWER SOUPS FOR A HEALTHY PROSTATE

Power food	What it does	Soup number
Brazil nuts	Rich in zinc, which helps combat prostate enlargement. Rich in selenium, which helps to prevent prostate cancer.	2
Fish	Rich in zinc. Also rich in selenium, which helps to prevent prostate cancer.	11, 36, 46, 53, 54, 55, 57, 60
Pumpkin seeds	Rich in zinc and in oils which help to balance male hormones	26
Soy foods: soy milk, tofu, soy flour, soy sauce, miso	Help to control prostate growth. Also help to prevent prostate cancer.	12, 33, 36, 39, 41, 44, 47, 51
Tomatoes and tomato purée	Rich in lycopene, which helps to prevent prostate cancer	8, 15, 17, 23, 26, 28, 43, 47, 57

AMAZING DISCOVERIES ABOUT FOOD AND HORMONES

2003 Research from the Cavale Blanche Hospital, Brest, France

Before three weeks of fish oil supplementation, volunteers placed under mental stress showed a fairly high heart rate and blood pressure. Adrenal hormone levels were also high. After three weeks of fish oil supplementation, all these measurements were significantly lower. The researchers concluded that fish oils can inhibit the adrenal activation caused by mental stress.

Delarue J. and colleagues. *Diabetes Metab.* 2003 Jun;29(3):289–95.

1994 Research from the Department of Nutrition, School of Public Health, University of North Carolina, USA

Low magnesium status increases the release of stress hormones, which in turn deplete magnesium levels. The hormones also stimulate the release of fatty acids. These complex with magnesium, making it less available for the body. All stress – whether exertion, heat, cold, trauma, pain, anxiety, excitement or even asthma attacks – increases the need for magnesium.

Seelig M.S. *J Am Coll Nutr* 1994.13(5):429–46.

1983 Research Reported in the *International Journal of Vitamin and Nutrition Research*

High-dose vitamin B_5 supplementation increases the excretion of ketosteroids in the urine. This is a sign that the adrenal glands are working better.

Fidanza A. Therapeutic action of pantothenic acid. *Int J Vit Nutr Res*, Suppl 24: In *Vitamins in Medicine: Recent therapeutic aspects*. A Hanck (Ed) 1983.

2002 Research from the Laboratory for Human Nutrition, Swiss Federal Institute of Technology, Zurich, Switzerland

Several minerals and trace elements, including iodine, iron, selenium and zinc, are essential for normal thyroid hormone metabolism. Deficiencies of these elements can impair thyroid function. A deficiency of both iron and iodine together is especially harmful. Supplementation with iodine is less effective when iron is deficient. Combined selenium and iodine deficiency is also highly detrimental. One task of selenium is to prevent the thyroid gland from absorbing excessive amounts of iodine. By controlling iodine absorption, selenium supplementation can lead to hypothyroidism when there is an iodine deficiency.

Zimmermann M.B. and colleagues. *Thyroid.* 2002 Oct;12(10):867–78.

1976 Research reported in *The Lancet*

Iodine deficiency seems to have a stimulatory effect on oestrogen production.

Stadel B.V. Dietary iodine and risk of breast, endometrial and ovarian cancer. *Lancet* 1976; 24 April:890–891.

1996 Research from the Department of Life Sciences and Chemistry, Roskilde University, Denmark

Cruciferous vegetables help the liver to metabolize oestrogen more efficiently.

Kall M.A. et al: Effects of dietary broccoli on human in vivo drug metabolizing enzymes: evaluation of caffeine, oestrone and chlorzoxazone metabolism. *Carcinogenesis* 17(4):793–9, 1996.

1994 Research from the Department of Medicine, University of Liege, Belgium

Magnesium deficiency results in impaired insulin secretion and reduces tissue sensitivity to insulin.

Lefebvre P.J. et al: Magnesium and glucose metabolism (in French). *Therapie* 1994;49(1):1–7.

2005 Research from the Sapporo Medical University School of Medicine, Japan

Recently, there have been reports that insulin resistance is linked with magnesium deficiency. Magnesium deficiency prevents receptors from taking up glucose. This makes the pancreas produce more insulin, but high levels of insulin encourage magnesium excretion, which further aggravates the problem.

Higashiura K. and colleagues. *Clin Calcium.* 2005 Feb;15(2):251–4.

1992 Research from the Department of Medicine, University of California, La Jolla, USA

Insulin resistance is a prominent feature in women with polycystic ovarian syndrome (PCOS). In this study, eight women with PCOS were compared with a control group of women without this condition. All members of the PCOS group had high insulin levels, especially when given sugar. All showed signs of insulin resistance, with cells failing to absorb glucose until blood levels of insulin reached eight times the norm.

Ciaraldi T.P., el-Roeiy A., Madar Z. et al. Cellular mechanisms of insulin resistance in polycystic ovarian syndrome. *J Clin Endocrinol Metab*1992;75:577–583.

2004 Research from the USDA Human Nutrition Research Center, Tufts University, Boston, USA.

Observational studies have found that diets rich in whole-grain foods reduce insulin resistance. The improved insulin sensitivity may be due in part to the magnesium and dietary fibre found in whole-grain foods. The researchers suggest that consuming whole-grain foods could help to treat insulin resistance.

McKeown N.M. *Nutr Rev.* 2004 Jul;62(7 Pt 1):286–91.

PART IV

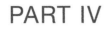

SOUP
RECIPES

FRUIT SOUPS

1	Apple, almond and cardamom soup with live yoghurt	LC
2	Avocado and banana soup with almonds and strawberries	(WF)
3	Baked fruit, cashew and cinnamon soup	LC, WF
4	Blackberry and vodka soup	GI
5	Dried fruit soup with pecans	LC
6	Peach and mango soup with coconut milk and yoghurt	LC, (WF)

SPECIAL SOUPS

7	Potage of celery and parsley (water release soup)	GI, WF
8	Rejuvenation soup	GI, WF

CABBAGE SOUPS

9	Basque cabbage and haricot bean soup	LC
10	Cabbage and ham soup with petits pois	GI
11	Spicy cabbage soup with cod and garlic	GI, (WF)
12	Thick and creamy cabbage soup with soft goat's cheese	GI, WF
13	Traditional Ukrainian borscht	GI

COLD SOUPS

14	Ajo blanco (Chilled garlic and almond soup)	GI
15	Avocado salsa soup	GI, LC
16	Chilled raspberry borscht	WF
17	Chilled tomato soup with cucumber and a hint of chilli	GI, LC, WF

STARTERS

18	Cream of asparagus soup	
19	French lettuce soup	GI, LC
20	French onion soup	GI, LC

THE BIG HEALTHY SOUP DIET

21	Healthy instant soup	GI, LC
22	Hungarian mushroom soup	GI
23	Italian tomato and parsley soup	GI, (WF)
24	Potage de Crécy	GI
25	Broad bean soup with apple and radish	LC, WF
26	Quick and easy cream of tomato soup	GI, LC
27	Quick and easy cream of vegetable soup	GI
28	Roasted Mediterranean vegetable soup	GI, LC, (WF)
29	Russian lemon soup	GI, (WF)
30	South Indian spicy sambhar soup	GI, LC, WF
31	Vichyssoise	
32	Watercress soup	WF

SUBSTANTIAL SOUPS ('ONE-POT MEALS')

33	Broccoli cream soup with Stilton cheese	GI
34	Brown lentil soup with roasted sweet peppers and apricots	GI, WF
35	Brussels butterbean bisque	GI, LC, (WF)

36	Butternut bisque with Cajun-style red mullet	GI, LC, WF
37	Carrot, chicken and sweetcorn spicy chowder	(WF)
38	Chinese egg and spring onion soup	
39	Chinese hot and sour soup	GI, LC
40	Cream of cauliflower soup	GI, LC, (WF)
41	Cream of mushroom soup with shiitake	GI, WF
42	German marrowfat pea soup with sausage	GI
43	Hungarian minestrone with shallots and brown beans	GI
44	Japanese buckwheat noodle soup	WF
45	Lemon dal soup	GI, LC, WF
46	Malaysian laksa	GI, (WF)
47	Mexican bean and lime soup with tofu	GI, LC, WF
48	Moroccan chickpea chorba	GI, WF
49	Mung bean soup with garlic and ginger	GI, LC, WF
50	Paraguayan zucchini soup with egg	GI
51	Potato and walnut pesto soup with tofu	WF
52	Red lentil and chestnut soup	GI, WF

53	Salmon and potato chunky chowder	GI
54	Scallop and potato chowder	GI, (WF)
55	Seafood bisque cooked French-style	GI, (WF)
56	Soupe à la courgette	GI, LC
57	Soupe de poisson (French fish soup)	GI, LC
58	Spinach and French lentil soup	GI, LC, WF
59	Sweet potato and groundnut soup	GI, (WF)
60	Thai shrimp noodle soup	
61	Thai tom kha gai (chicken and vegetable) soup	GI, LC

Key

GI	Compatible with low-glycaemic index diets
LC	Compatible with low-carbohydrate diets
WF	Compatible with the Waterfall Diet
(WF)	Compatible with the Waterfall Diet if non-dairy options and unsalted stock are used

---

Note: in these recipes, 1 cup is equal to 300 ml (10 fl oz or half a pint).

FRUIT SOUPS

1. Apple, almond and cardamom soup with live yoghurt

2 SERVINGS

4 large sweet apples, peeled, cored and cut into chunks*

2 tbsp ground almonds (almond flour)

2 tbsp unsalted butter†

4 tbsp plain live, organic yoghurt§

Apple or pear juice

1 cardamom pod

Garnish: strands of orange and lemon zest

* Use a variety with a good flavour, such as Cox's.

† For the 4-day detox, use sunflower oil instead.

§ For the 4-day detox, use only sheep's, goat's or soy yoghurt.

Remove the husk from the cardamom pod, and grind the seeds with a mortar and pestle.

Melt the butter in a saucepan over a low heat, stir in the ground cardamom then add the apple pieces and stir-fry for two minutes. Now add the ground almonds and then pour in enough apple or pear juice to cover the contents of the pan. Bring to simmering point then place a lid on the pan and leave to simmer gently for 20 minutes.

Remove from the heat and whizz with a hand blender until smooth. Serve warm, with a swirl of yoghurt. Garnish with strands of orange and lemon zest.

What it's good for

This soup is ideal for breakfast. Rich in vitamin C and pectin, but providing only about 50 calories each, apples are a great aid to losing weight, especially when cooked and eaten warm, when they are so much more filling. Cooking breaks down tough cellulose in plant foods, allowing better digestion.

Cardamom is a very complementary spice for apples, and almonds not only give this soup some protein, but are also rich in calcium, magnesium, zinc and monounsaturated oils. LDL (bad) cholesterol can be reduced by consuming almonds regularly. Yoghurt provides beneficial 'friendly' bacteria.

2. Avocado and banana soup with almonds and strawberries

2–4 SERVINGS

1 avocado pear, peeled and roughly diced
1 banana, cut into chunks
600 ml/1 pint/2 cups dairy or soy milk
110 g/¼ lb fresh strawberries, chopped
1 small carton plain live, organic dairy or soy yoghurt
1 tbsp ground almonds (almond flour)*
1 tbsp lemon juice
Garnish: a sprig of fresh mint

* Instead of almonds you could use Brazil nuts. Prepare Brazil nuts by grating them with a drum grater (a grater with a handle that you turn).

Place the avocado, banana, lemon juice, yoghurt, ground almonds and milk in a blender and whizz until smooth. Place the chopped strawberries in a serving dish and pour the avocado mixture over them. Decorate with a sprig of mint.

The flavour and colour of avocado begin to break down when it is liquidized, so this soup needs to be consumed immediately.

You could also make this into a breakfast 'smoothie' by leaving out the strawberries or whizzing them into the other ingredients.

What it's good for

Avocado pears are extremely nutritious, rich in protein, polyunsaturated and monounsaturated oils, vitamin B6 and other B-vitamins, vitamin E, iron and copper. They provide three times as much potassium as bananas. The ground almonds and yoghurt add further protein, calcium, magnesium and other minerals to this dish. Live yoghurt has anti-cancer properties and is a useful remedy for diarrhoea caused by food poisoning bacteria.

According to recent research from the University of Illinois, straw-berries contain phytonutrients with anti-inflammatory powers similar to those of anti-arthritis medicines. They can also help to prevent damage to cells from cancer-causing chemicals, and inhibit the development of cancers. Strawberries may even help to prevent Alzheimer's disease and senility.

Brazil nuts are rich in zinc, copper and methionine. In the UK, New Zealand and other countries with low levels of selenium in the soil, they are the only good plant source of the essential mineral selenium.

3. Baked fruit, cashew and cinnamon soup

1 SERVING

225 g/8 oz dark red or purple fruits (e.g. blueberries, bilberries,
   blackberries, black cherries, plums)*
1 generous handful raw cashew nuts
70 ml/3 fl oz/¼ cup red grape juice
½ tsp ground cinnamon

* Fresh fruit is best, but you can use frozen if necessary

Preheat the oven to 180°C/350°F/Gas Mark 4. If using fresh fruit, rinse it and mop dry with a kitchen towel.

Remove any stones from cherries, plums etc. Place the fruit in a lidded oven-proof dish and bake for 20 minutes until tender and juicy. Meanwhile, rinse the cashew nuts and dry them with a kitchen towel or absorbent paper. (This is to remove powdery deposits which affect their flavour.) Put the nuts on a baking tray and place them in the oven with the fruit, for a maximum of five minutes. Keep an eye on the nuts. The aim is not to brown them, only to bring out their flavour. Remove them and allow to cool.

When the fruit is ready, put it in a shallow serving dish and sprinkle with cinnamon. Spoon the grape juice over the top, and finally the cashew nuts.

What it's good for

Dark-red and purple fruits are rich in flavonoids which, if eaten regularly, help to prevent small blood vessels from leaking water and protein into surrounding tissues. This makes these fruits especially useful in combating water retention. They act in a similar way to the herb ginkgo biloba, which, by strengthening the capillaries in the brain, has been shown to help prevent Alzheimer's disease and senility. By helping to maintain the integrity of the microcirculation, these flavonoid-rich foods can also benefit eyesight and hearing and help to prevent varicose veins.

Most of us are used to eating salted cashew nuts and do not realize how deliciously sweet these nuts are in their natural state. Raw cashews are low in oil and rich in potassium and magnesium, iron and zinc. Always wash raw cashews before use as they can develop a little mould, which may affect their flavour.

4. Blackberry and vodka soup

450 g/1 lb/4 scant cups fresh or frozen blackberries
1 cup red grape juice
2 tbsp vodka
2 rounded tsp powdered arrowroot
Garnish: a spoonful of Greek yoghurt and a sprig of mint

Put the blackberries in a saucepan with the grape juice. Put a lid on the pan, bring to the boil and simmer over a very low heat until tender and juicy (two to five minutes if fresh and a little longer if frozen).

Put the arrowroot powder in a small bowl and stir in 2 tbsp water to make a smooth paste. Stir this paste into the blackberries, and keep stirring until the mixture thickens. Stir in the vodka.

Serve warm or cold with a spoonful of Greek yoghurt in the centre, decorated with a sprig of mint.

Variations

Using the same method, this soup can also be made with blueberries, bilberries and black cherries, all of which have similar nutritional properties.

What it's good for

Vodka? Well they say a little of what you fancy does you good, and in this case a little goes a long way.

Dark-red and purple fruits are rich in flavonoids, which, if eaten regularly, help to prevent small blood vessels from leaking water and protein into surrounding tissues. This makes these fruits especially useful in combating water retention. They act in a similar way to the herb ginkgo biloba, which, by strengthening the capillaries in the brain, has been shown to help prevent Alzheimer's disease and senility. By helping to maintain the integrity of the microcirculation, these flavonoid-rich foods can also benefit eyesight and hearing and help to prevent varicose veins.

5. Dried fruit soup with pecans

8 dried prunes

8 dried apricots*

2 tbsp raisins

2 large, sweet apples, peeled, cored and cut into chunks

1 cup apple or white grape juice

4 tbsp yoghurt†

Half a cup of pecan nuts, chopped

2 tbsp unsalted butter

1 pinch cinnamon

* Use unsulphured apricots if possible. These are dark-brown in colour, whereas the orange variety has been treated with preservatives that can irritate the digestive system.

† For the 4-day detox, use only sheep's, goat's or soy yoghurt.

Heat the butter in a saucepan over a medium heat, stir in the cinnamon, then add the apples and stir-fry for two minutes until beginning to soften. Add the prunes, dried apricots and raisins, then pour in the juice. Place a lid on the pan, bring to the boil, and simmer gently for 10 minutes. Serve warm, topped with a spoonful of yoghurt and sprinkled with chopped pecans.

What it's good for

Dried fruit makes a good breakfast and is rich in fibre, potassium and minerals. Pecans add their own delicious sweetness to this dish, as well as protein and essential polyunsaturated oils. They are one of the best natural sources of vitamin B6. Yoghurt is a good source of beneficial 'friendly' bacteria.

By serving this soup warm for breakfast, you avoid chilling your digestive system. This not only helps you digest your food better but also keeps your appetite satisfied for longer.

If you prefer to serve this soup as a cold dessert, use groundnut oil instead of butter.

6. Peach and mango soup with coconut milk and yoghurt

6 SERVINGS

4 large, juicy peaches*

1 ripe mango, peeled

1 can (400 ml/14 fl oz) coconut milk†

1 small carton (½ cup) plain dairy or soy yoghurt

2 pieces of stem ginger (from a jar, in syrup), drained and finely
   shredded

1 tbsp syrup from the jar of stem ginger

Garnish: a sprig of fresh mint

* Truly ripe peaches should drip juice when cut with a knife. This recipe can also be made with canned peaches.

† Coconut milk is juice extracted from grated fresh coconut. (The liquid that pours out when you crack open a coconut is called coconut water.) The best brands of coconut milk often come from health-food or Asian shops, and consist of 55 per cent coconut extract with 45 per cent water. Stabilizers, thickeners or other additives are not necessary.

Immerse the can of coconut milk in a bowl of hot water to help melt the coconut oils.

Meanwhile, using a sharp knife, cut all the way through the mango lengthwise on either side of the large, flat stone in the centre, cutting as close to the stone as you can to remove the flesh. Do the same on the other side. Cut the flesh into small dice.

Stone the peaches, chop them roughly and place in a blender. If the peaches are hard, place the pieces in a small saucepan, add half a cup of water, cover the pan and simmer for 20 minutes until softened. Allow to cool, then drain and place in the blender.

Remove the can of coconut milk from the hot water and shake thoroughly for about 10 seconds. Open the can, and add the contents to the blender. Add the yoghurt and the ginger syrup. Whizz until smooth and creamy.

Pour into a bowl and stir in the diced mango and shredded stem ginger. Serve garnished with a sprig of fresh mint.

Variation

Make this into a breakfast 'smoothie' by simply liquidizing all the ingredients. Or, for extra vitamin C, use diced kiwi fruit instead of mango.

Note: This soup should not be chilled.

What it's good for

Peaches and mangoes are a good source of vitamin C and carotene antioxidants. Coconut milk contains beneficial oils which have been found to combat viruses. Dairy yoghurt is a good source of calcium plus lots of other nutrients and friendly bacteria.

SPECIAL SOUPS

7. Potage of celery and parsley (Water release soup)

4 SERVINGS

1 head of celery, roughly chopped

1 head of celery, juiced*

850 ml/1½ pints/3 cups water or broad bean stock[†]

1 medium potato, diced

1 large onion, roughly chopped

1 can of broad beans (fava beans), rinsed and drained[§]

2 tbsp flax oil

4 tbsp sunflower seeds

1 large handful fresh parsley leaves, finely chopped

Stalks from the parsley, roughly chopped

2 tbsp soy cream

Black pepper

* To make celery juice you need a juice extractor. If you do not have one, you can use an extra cup of water instead, but the soup will not be as effective.

[†] Boil cleaned, chopped broad bean pods in the water for 30 minutes and then strain.

[§] When fresh broad beans are in season, you can use a cupful of these instead. After adding them, just bring the soup back to a gentle simmer and cook for 8–10 minutes or until tender.

Put the water or stock and celery juice, diced potato, sunflower seeds, chopped celery, onion and parsley stalks in a covered saucepan over a high heat, and bring to the boil. Then reduce the heat to a gentle simmer and leave to cook for 25 minutes or until the potatoes and celery are tender.

Remove from the heat and liquidize with a hand blender. Then add the broad beans and return the pan to a gentle simmer for two minutes until the beans are heated through. If using fresh broad beans, cook them for 5–10 minutes until tender.

Just before serving, stir in the soy cream, flax oil and chopped parsley leaves and season with black pepper. Do not add salt to this soup.

What it's good for

Celery and parsley help your immune system to break down protein particles which have leaked into your tissue spaces, and lie there attracting water retention. Once the particles have been removed, the excess water can drain away. These two foods also act as natural, gentle diuretics, helping your kidneys to excrete the fluid. Unlike pharmaceutical drugs, they help to replace the nutrients that diuretics remove from your body.

The sunflower seeds in this recipe help to contribute useful amino acids such as methionine and tryptophan.

In Oriental medicine, stock made from broad bean pods is considered very helpful for removing water retention.

8. Rejuvenation soup

1 carcass from an organic chicken or other organically-raised
    poultry*

The bird's giblets (liver, neck and heart)

1.7 litres/3 pints/6 cups water

2 large handfuls of dark green leaves, shredded[†]

2 carrots, sliced

2 tomatoes, roughly chopped

2 tbsp brown rice

1 medium onion, chopped

1 tbsp brown rice miso

4 cloves of garlic, crushed

A few shreds of wakame seaweed

1 thumb-sized piece of ginger, peeled and grated

The juice of half a lemon

1 tbsp extra-virgin olive oil

Cayenne pepper to taste

Low-sodium salt

½ tsp turmeric (optional)

SPECIAL EQUIPMENT

A pressure cooker

* For example, the remains of a roast chicken or duck, or the carcass left after filleting a chicken. Your butcher may be able to supply this.

[†] Use the darkest green you can find: spring (collard) greens, kale, watercress, Brussels sprout tops or outer leaves of Savoy cabbage are all suitable.

Put the rice to soak in a cup of water. Cut any greenish-yellow marks off the liver (these are bitter). Cut up or break up the carcass so that the bones will take up as little space as possible in a pan. Put the bones in a pressure cooker together with the giblets and water and ensure they are covered with water. Bring to full steam and cook for 25 minutes. Allow to cool naturally, then strain the stock through a sieve into a large saucepan. Drain the rice and add to the pan. Add the miso and stir to dissolve, then add the vegetables and other ingredients.

Use your hands to pick the remains of any meat on the carcass, and put them in the saucepan. Crumble the liver with your fingers, or pound it to a paste in a mortar and pestle. Thinly slice the heart. Look for any bones which have become very soft, and pound one of these in a mortar and pestle until you have a teaspoon of paste. Stir these ingredients into the liquid. Discard the remains of the carcass. You can add the optional turmeric at this stage. It is a very healthy ingredient, but be prepared for it to turn the soup yellow!

Now bring the pan to the boil, cover it and simmer for 40 minutes. Taste the soup and add a little salt if necessary. Add a little more cayenne pepper if you think it could do with a touch more zing.

What it's good for

This soup is truly loaded with health-giving ingredients and is a great way to use the giblets from a chicken or duck, plus the bones which normally get thrown away. In effect, you are getting a couple more meals out of the bird. Liver is rich in protein, vitamin A, folic acid, iron, copper, zinc and B-vitamins. Bones are rich in calcium, magnesium and many other minerals, as well as glycine, which helps your liver to process toxins. The joints release glucosamine, which helps to nourish your own joints. Chilli pepper and ginger warm the circulation and aid blood flow. Seaweed provides precious iodine. With the B-vitamins in the brown rice and miso, special sulphur compounds in the garlic and onions, and the antioxidants in the carrots and dark green leaves, eating this soup regularly could seriously rejuvenate you! See page 237 for the health benefits of turmeric.

CABBAGE SOUPS

The original cabbage soup diet was based on a recipe that consisted of boiling together the following ingredients: water, cabbage, onion, canned tomatoes, green peppers, carrots, green beans, celery, dry onion soup powder, black pepper, plus herbs and vinegar to taste.

There really is nothing magical about these ingredients, so it is quite likely that the success of the diet lay mainly in the fact that it was soup. As research has shown, incorporating liquid with food seems to have significant appetite-calming effects.

Maybe some people are happy to eat the same cabbage soup recipe day after day. But if you are not, here are five more cabbage soup recipes for you to enjoy and at the same time to reap all the health benefits of cabbage!

What it's good for

Cabbage helps your liver to process toxins and hormone residues into harmless substances. It is especially good for women with health problems associated with high oestrogen levels. Cabbage is also rich in a powerful antioxidant flavonoid known as quercetin, which has been found to help combat viruses and prevent cataracts and allergic problems. Use the darkest-green cabbage you can find. Savoy cabbage (the dark-green crinkly variety) is especially good.

Basque cabbage and haricot bean soup

Because of their salt, red meat and animal fat content, it is not healthy to eat bacon, chorizo sausage or pancetta every day, but a little goes a long way, and these ingredients are useful to flavour what might otherwise be quite a bland soup.

½ medium green cabbage, shredded

2 cups cooked haricot beans*

225 g/8 oz chorizo sausage, cut into chunks†

1 medium onion, cut in half lengthwise then thinly sliced

2 garlic cloves, crushed

4 tbsp olive oil

Caraway or fennel seeds

Low-sodium salt and freshly ground black pepper

Boiling water

* See page 272 for preparing pulses (legumes) or use canned beans that have been rinsed and drained.

† Some varieties are quite fiery, so ask before you buy!

Soften the onion in the olive oil over a medium heat in a large saucepan. Stir in the cabbage, then add about one cup of boiling water. Cover the pan and bring to the boil. Cook the cabbage over a medium heat for five minutes, stirring occasionally. The cabbage should now be collapsed and beginning to get tender.

Using a fork, roughly mash half of the beans, which will help to thicken the soup.

Add the garlic, beans, sausage chunks and caraway seeds to the pan, stir well, and pour in just enough boiling water almost to cover the contents of the pan. Bring to the boil and simmer gently for 40 minutes. Taste the soup and add a little salt and freshly ground black pepper (if needed) before serving.

Variations

This dish (like most of the soups in this book which require lengthy simmering) can also be cooked in a 'slow cooker'. Simply place the soup in the slow cooker when it gets to the simmering stage, and leave it to cook while you go out for the day. It will be delicious and ready to eat when you get home.

You can also use pancetta instead of chorizo. While the soup is cooking, cut 50 g/2 oz pancetta or thick-cut bacon into small cubes and fry in a frying pan (skillet) until beginning to get crispy. Stir these into the soup five minutes before serving.

Traditional peasant version

Cover a joint of uncooked ham, bacon or gammon with water in a soup pan and boil for two hours or until cooked through. Remove the joint and set aside to rest. Cook the soup using the method above, replacing the boiling water with broth from boiling the bacon. When the soup is ready, carve the bacon into portions, place them in individual bowls and pour the soup over the top.

10. Cabbage and ham soup with petits pois

4 SERVINGS

¼ cabbage, chopped
1.2 litres/2 pints/4 cups chicken or vegetable stock (broth)
1 large potato, peeled and cut into chunks
1 cup fresh or frozen (defrosted) petits pois
225 g/8 oz cooked ham, diced
1 onion, chopped
2 tbsp olive oil
Low-sodium salt and freshly ground black pepper
Garnish: a sprig of mint

Heat the olive oil in a large saucepan. Add the onion and stir-fry over a medium heat for a few minutes to soften. Add the potato chunks, cabbage and stock and bring to the boil. Reduce the heat and simmer gently for 30 minutes until the ingredients are tender. Using a hand blender, whizz until smooth then return to the heat and add the ham and petits pois. Bring to simmering point and simmer gently for two minutes. Taste the soup and add a little salt if necessary. (You may not need any if you used a stock cube, and ham itself is quite salty.) Before serving, season with freshly ground black pepper and garnish with a sprig of mint.

Variation

This soup can be made with a cup of diced carrots instead of peas. Dice the carrots quite small so that the pieces will not take too long to become tender. Or you could try adding black-eyed beans (rinsed and drained) from a can. As they are already cooked, these will only need a couple of minutes' simmering time.

11. Spicy cabbage soup with cod and garlic

1 small to medium green cabbage*
225 g/8 oz fresh cod (or other white fish) fillets
600 ml/1 pint/2 cups vegetable stock (broth)
½ cup uncooked or 1 cup cooked brown rice
1 medium onion
4 cloves garlic
2 red chilli peppers†
1 thumb-sized piece of fresh ginger
4 tbsp olive oil
Low-sodium salt
Boiling water

* The Savoy cabbage with its dark-green, crinkly leaves is good for this soup.

† Use a medium-sized (medium-hot) variety. The smaller the chilli, the hotter it is.

If using uncooked brown rice, start by cooking this separately. Put the rice in a small pan with just over twice its volume of boiling water. Bring to the boil, put a lid on the pan and simmer gently for 20–25 minutes until tender. If any excess liquid remains, drain it away. Put the rice in a warm oven to keep hot.

Meanwhile, prepare the vegetables. Finely shred the cabbage. Cut the onion in half lengthwise then slice it thinly lengthwise. Crush or finely grate the garlic. Peel and grate the ginger. Deseed and finely chop the chilli peppers. Cut the fish into bite-sized chunks.

Using a large, heavy-bottomed saucepan, fry the onion in the olive oil over a medium heat until tender but not brown. Stir in the chilli, ginger and garlic, followed by the shredded cabbage. Add a cup of hot water. Cover the pan, bring it to the boil then allow the cabbage to steam vigorously for five minutes, stirring occasionally. Ensure it does not boil dry, and add more water if necessary.

When the cabbage has collapsed, stir in the stock plus enough boiling water to cover the contents of the pan. Bring to the boil, replace the lid, then simmer gently for 30 minutes. Stir in the chunks of fish and simmer for a further five minutes or until the fish is opaque and flakes easily. Taste the soup and add a little salt if necessary. (You may not need any if you used a stock cube.)

Spoon the cooked rice into a serving dish and ladle the soup over it.

12. Thick and creamy cabbage soup with soft goat's cheese

4 SERVINGS

Half a medium-sized white cabbage, shredded

1.2 litres/2 pints/4 cups dairy or soy milk

2 medium potatoes*

110 g/4 oz soft goat's cheese

1 slightly rounded tbsp arrowroot powder

2 cloves garlic, crushed

2 bay leaves

Grated nutmeg

Low-sodium salt and freshly ground black pepper

Garnish: fresh chives

* Use a waxy variety such as Cara or Desirée

Put the shredded cabbage in a large saucepan with one cup of water. Bring to the boil, cover the pan tightly, then continue to boil over a medium heat for five minutes or until the cabbage has begun to soften and collapse. (Ensure the pan does not boil dry.)

Stir in the bay leaves, garlic and nutmeg, followed by the milk plus, if necessary, some more water to cover the cabbage. Return to the boil, then turn down the heat to its lowest setting and simmer very gently for one hour, stirring from time to time.

While this is happening, boil the potatoes in their jackets until tender all the way through when tested with a knife (about 40 minutes after the water comes to the boil). Drain and plunge into a sink of cold water for a few minutes until they have cooled down enough to handle them. Drain the potatoes again and peel them, using a small sharp knife. Put to one side.

Five minutes before the end of the cooking time, mix the arrowroot in a small bowl with a few tablespoons of water until you have a runny paste. Pour this paste into the saucepan and keep stirring the soup until it thickens a little.

At the end of the cooking time, take the pan off the heat, stir the soft goat's cheese into the pan, and keep stirring until it has all melted. Now cut the potatoes into bite-sized pieces, fold the potato pieces into the soup and gently warm through but do not allow to boil. Taste the soup and add a little salt if necessary. Season with freshly ground black pepper and garnish with fresh chives.

13. Traditional Ukrainian borscht

600 ml/1 pint/2 cups chicken or vegetable stock (broth)

Half a medium green cabbage, coarsely shredded

3 medium potatoes, cut into four lengthwise, then thinly sliced

3 medium beetroot (beets), boiled whole, peeled, cooled and
   coarsely grated

2 medium carrots, coarsely grated

1 medium onion

1 small can tomato purée (paste)

4 tbsp olive oil

Low-sodium salt and freshly ground black pepper

Boiling water

Garnish: sour cream and fresh chopped chives

Put the potatoes and shredded cabbage in a large saucepan and press down. Pour in the stock plus just enough water to barely cover the ingredients, and bring to the boil. Simmer with the lid on for 15 minutes, then add the grated carrot and simmer for a further five minutes or until the ingredients are tender.

Meanwhile cut the onion into eight pieces and process in a food processor with the 'S' blade, until very finely chopped. Heat the oil in a stir-fry pan or sauté pan, and stir the onion mixture over a medium heat until softened but not brown.

When the cabbage, potato and carrot are tender, stir in the tomato purée then add the softened onion and olive oil, followed by the grated beetroot and black pepper. Taste the soup and add a little salt if necessary. (You may not need any if you used a stock cube.) Gently heat through, then serve in bowls topped with a spoonful of sour cream and some fresh chopped chives.

What it's good for

I was given this recipe when I visited the Ukraine, where it forms part of the staple diet. The Ukrainians would normally use sunflower oil, but I have replaced this with olive oil, which is more stable when heated. Beetroot is a wonderful herb-like food which stimulates your liver cells, and is one of the richest plant sources of iron in a well-assimilated form.

It is also traditional to add a little shredded chicken to Ukrainian borscht. I have left this out because I think the soup is better without it; but you could add a little if you want to increase the protein content.

COLD SOUPS

14. Ajo blanco
(Chilled garlic and almond soup)

4 SERVINGS

200 g/7 oz/1 cup ground almonds*

2 garlic cloves, chopped

2 apples, peeled, cored and chopped†

100 ml/3 fl oz/⅓ cup extra-virgin olive oil

A loaf of stale French bread, sliced, with crusts removed

2 tsp apple cider vinegar

Low-sodium salt

A jug of iced or chilled water

Garnish: white grapes

* You get a better flavour if you buy blanched almonds and grind them yourself in a food processor, but you will need to pass the soup through a sieve before serving to remove any large particles.

† Choose a variety with a good flavour, such as Cox's.

Put the chopped apples in a small saucepan with a few tablespoons of water and cook over a low heat until soft and mushy (5–10 minutes). Allow to cool completely. Put the bread in a bowl and sprinkle in enough iced water to soften it thoroughly.

Put the ground almonds, bread, garlic, apple vinegar, salt and olive oil in a liquidizer and top up with just enough water to allow the blender to run smoothly. Blend until smooth, then test the consistency with a teaspoon. Add chilled water a little at a time until you obtain the consistency of pouring cream.

This soup can be served immediately, but can also be kept in the fridge for a few hours before serving, and this reduces the rawness of the garlic flavour. Ajo blanco is traditionally served garnished with white grapes.

What it's good for

If you are a garlic lover, you will adore this ancient Spanish recipe, which looks as if it has been made with lavish amounts of cream! The use of bread as a thickener does not sound appetizing, but you really will be surprised at the result, and the soup is wonderfully quick and simple to make.

Ajo blanco is not normally made with apples, but I have included some here as they provide extra nutrition, and their flavour really adds something to this recipe. Raw garlic has good antifungal and antibacterial properties, and almonds are a rich source of calcium, magnesium and zinc. LDL (bad) cholesterol can be reduced by consuming almonds regularly. Both almonds and olive oil provide healthy monounsaturated oils, and extra-virgin olive oil is rich in antioxidants.

15. Avocado salsa soup

4 ripe avocados
600 ml/1 pint/2 cups water
1 x 200 g carton (⅔ cup) low-fat fromage frais
1 small onion, diced
2 tomatoes, skinned*
Juice of 1 lime
1 small green chilli pepper, deseeded and roughly chopped
1 tbsp extra-virgin olive oil
½ tsp dried garlic granules
Low-sodium salt and freshly ground black pepper
Garnish: chopped tomato and thinly sliced spring onion

* To skin tomatoes, leave them in a bowl of boiling water for 60 seconds, then drain and rinse with cold water. Use a sharp knife to remove the peel, which should come off easily.

Place the water in a blender with the lime juice, fromage frais, diced onion, chilli, garlic granules, olive oil and a pinch of salt. Cut the skinned tomatoes in half and scoop out the seeds into a small bowl. Press the water from the tomato pulp through a fine sieve into the blender and discard the seeds. Finely dice the tomato flesh and reserve to one side.

Cut the avocados in half, discard the stones, scoop out the flesh and add it to the blender. Whizz until smooth and creamy. Serve immediately, topped with a spoonful of diced tomato and sprinkled with sliced spring onions. Season with freshly ground black pepper. This dish will not keep, as the avocados will discolour and lose their flavour.

What it's good for

Avocado pears are extremely nutritious, rich in protein, polyunsaturated and monounsaturated oils, vitamin B6 and other B-vitamins, vitamin E, iron and copper. They provide three times as much potassium as bananas. Fromage frais is a good source of calcium and protein. Raw onion (in juice form) is a traditional remedy for the treatment of burns. In liquidized form, as in this recipe, it has soothing and healing properties for the intestines.

16. Chilled raspberry borscht

450 g/1 lb cooked beetroots (beets), cut roughly into chunks*

275 ml/½ pint/1 cup beetroot (beet) juice†

110 g/¼ lb/½ cup fresh raspberries

1 medium red onion, cut roughly into chunks

Fresh lemon juice to taste

1 tbsp balsamic vinegar

Sour cream

Garnish: strands of lemon and orange zest

* Alternatively, if you can find fresh beetroots, cook them yourself. Trim and scrub the raw beetroots and place whole in a saucepan with enough water to cover them. Place a lid on the pan, bring to the boil and simmer until tender (about 30–45 minutes, depending on the size). Drain, allow to cool, then peel and cut roughly into chunks.

† Available from health-food stores.

Place the beetroot pieces, beetroot juice, raspberries, onion chunks and balsamic vinegar in a blender and whizz until smooth. Pass through a sieve to remove the raspberry seeds. Taste the mixture, then stir in the lemon juice a few drops at a time until you get the balance you prefer, between the sweetness of the beetroot and the tanginess of the lemon juice. If you find the soup too thick, add a little more beetroot juice.

Chill the soup in the refrigerator. Serve with a spoonful of sour cream and garnish with strands of lemon and orange zest. This soup can also be served warm. It does not need any salt, but if you wish you can taste it and add a little at the last minute.

What it's good for

Beetroot is a wonderful herb-like food which stimulates your liver cells, and is one of the richest plant sources of iron in a well-assimilated form. Raspberries, like other dark red, blue or purple berries, are rich in a variety of cancer-preventing compounds such as ellagic acid and anthocyanidins.

17. Chilled tomato soup with cucumber and a hint of chilli

4 SERVINGS

1 litre/1¾ pints/3½ cups fresh tomato juice from a carton

2 large fresh tomatoes, skinned and diced*

1 cucumber

1 sweet (bell) pepper – red, yellow or orange in colour

1 spring onion (scallion), roughly chopped

4 tbsp extra-virgin olive oil

1 tsp capers

1 clove of garlic, crushed

A few drops of Tabasco sauce

Ice cubes

* To skin tomatoes, leave them in a bowl of boiling water for 60 seconds, then drain and rinse with cold water. Use a sharp knife to remove the peel, which should come off easily.

Reserve half of the cucumber and cut into tiny dice. Roughly chop the rest of the cucumber and place in a blender. After removing the stalk and seeds, do the same with the pepper. Add the tomato juice, crushed garlic, olive oil, spring onion, capers and Tabasco sauce to the blender, then whizz until you obtain a smooth consistency. Pour into a bowl and stir in the chopped tomatoes with their juice. Cover the bowl and chill thoroughly in the refrigerator. Just before serving, stir again and add ice cubes. Serve the diced cucumber and pepper separately, to be spooned into the soup. If you wish to add some salt, taste the soup and add it at the last minute.

What it's good for

Although it uses ready-made tomato juice, the natural deep-red colour of the tomatoes chosen for such products makes them healthy (but watch out for the salt content). The red colour is a pigment known as lycopene, and is a powerful antioxidant. Population studies suggest that people who consume lots of lycopene-rich foods have a lower risk of not only prostate cancer, but also cancer of the cervix, skin, bladder, breast, lung and digestive tract. The redder the tomato, the more lycopene it contains. The tomato is also an excellent source of folic acid, vitamin C and potassium.

Cucumber juice is a soothing traditional remedy for cystitis, and is said to help combat intestinal parasites such as worms. Cucumber is a good source of the bone-building mineral silicon.

STARTERS

18. Cream of asparagus soup

2 SERVINGS

Approx. 225 g/8 oz asparagus spears, washed
600 ml/1 pint/2 cups hot chicken or vegetable stock (broth)
1 medium onion, diced*
1 small to medium potato, diced
1 level tbsp rice or wheat flour
1 tbsp butter
1 tbsp cream
Low-sodium salt and freshly ground black pepper

* Avoid using red onions for this recipe, as they will affect the colour

Using your fingers, snap off and discard the woody part of the aspara-gus spears. Cut the spears roughly into 1 cm/$\frac{1}{2}$ inch segments. Melt the butter in a large saucepan over a medium heat. Add the chopped onion and stir-fry for a minute or two until beginning to soften. Sprin-kle with the flour and stir for 1–2 minutes, then pour about a cupful of the hot stock into the pan and keep stirring until the mixture begins to thicken. Stir in the rest of the stock, plus the potato, and bring to sim-mering point. Reduce the heat and simmer for 20 minutes. Now add the asparagus and cook for 10 minutes more.

Using a hand blender, whizz the soup until smooth, then return it to the saucepan and stir in the cream. Taste the soup and add a little salt if necessary (you may not need any if you used a stock cube) then gently heat through for a few minutes over a low heat and serve sea-soned with freshly ground black pepper.

What it's good for

It seems a shame to prepare asparagus in any other way than at its most simple and delicious. A little butter and cream go a long way in this dish.

Asparagus was in fact used medicinally long before it was eaten as a vegetable. It contains asparagine, which has diuretic properties, and is said to be able to break up crystals of uric and oxalic acids, thus helping to prevent both gout and kidney stones. Asparagus is also a source of aspartic acid, which helps to break down harmful ammonia in our bodies.

19. French lettuce soup

1–2 SERVINGS

1 head of cos or Romaine lettuce or 4 heads of the miniature
  variety (known as Little Gem)
275 ml/½ pint/1 cup vegetable stock (broth)
2 tbsp dairy or soy cream
2 tbsp butter
2 tbsp finely grated Emmenthal or Gruyère cheese
Fresh chives, chopped
Low-sodium salt and freshly ground black pepper

Keeping the lettuce whole, wash it and leave it upside down in a colander to drain for 10 minutes. Mop away any remaining moisture with a kitchen towel. Trim the stem of the lettuce, then cut the lettuce crosswise into rounds with a thickness of 5 cm/2 inches.

Melt the butter in a deep sauté pan over a medium heat. Carefully place the lettuce rounds side by side in a single layer in the pan and fry over a medium to high heat for two minutes or until the bottom of the lettuce is beginning to brown. Now add the stock, cover the pan and leave to simmer gently for 15 minutes or until all the lettuce pieces are tender. Using a spatula, transfer the lettuce pieces to a serving bowl, stir the cream into the juices in the pan, then pour them over the lettuce. Taste the liquid and add a little salt if necessary (you may not need any if you used a stock cube). Season with freshly ground black pepper and sprinkle with cheese and fresh chopped chives.

What it's good for

This soup provides no more calories than a green salad with mayonnaise and a little cheese, yet it is so much more satisfying! You may think of lettuce as a salad ingredient, but it is also a leafy green vegetable and is delicious when cooked. Like other leafy greens, it supplies magnesium, folic acid and other important nutrients. The sap of wild lettuce is rich in a substance related to opium, which can help you sleep. The sap is mainly in the root of the plant, but if you have trouble sleeping, this may be a good soup to eat before going to bed!

20. French onion soup

2–3 SERVINGS

4 large red onions, peeled, cut in half lengthwise then thinly sliced
lengthwise
2 tbsp olive oil
600 ml/1 pint/2 cups boiling water
70 ml/3 fl oz/¼ cup red wine
1 tbsp brown rice miso
1 tsp fresh chopped or ½ tsp dried thyme or marjoram
Low-sodium salt and freshly ground black pepper
Optional: French bread and Gruyère or Emmenthal cheese

Heat the oil in a large, shallow saucepan over a medium to high heat, then add the onions and stir-fry for about 20 minutes until beginning to caramelize. Add the water and red wine followed by the miso and thyme or marjoram. Stir well to dissolve the miso. Bring the liquid back to the boil, cover, and simmer over a low heat for 30 minutes. Check the consistency and add a little boiling water if it is too thick. Taste the soup and add a little salt if necessary (miso already contains salt). Season with freshly ground black pepper before serving.

Optional

Toast (on one side only) two slices of French baguette per serving. Sprinkle the toasted side with grated Gruyère or Emmenthal cheese and place under the grill (broiler) until melted. Put at the base of the serving bowl and pour the soup over the top.

What it's good for

Miso, olive oil and parsley make this an extra-healthy version of French onion soup. Miso is a Japanese flavouring used to make soup. Rich in B-vitamins and made from fermented soybeans, it is considered one of Japan's premier health foods. The therapeutic value of the humble onion is often forgotten in favour of its famous cousin garlic. Onions are a rich source of the anti-allergy flavonoid quercetin. Quercetin can inhibit the release of histamine, the cause of allergic symptoms, inflammation and asthma attacks. Quercetin has also been investigated for its virus-fighting properties. The colour in red onions is a natural pigment known as anthocyanin, which is a good antioxidant.

21. Healthy instant soup

1 tsp brown rice miso
1 tbsp thinly sliced spring onion (scallion)
A few shreds of dried seaweed*
Boiling water

* Health-food stores now sell many different types of dried seaweed. You can
experiment with any of these. The variety traditionally used in miso soup is known
as kombu.

Fill a large cup or mug with boiling water and add the miso, stirring
until it has thoroughly dissolved. Add the spring onion and seaweed
and leave to steep for a few minutes, after which it is ready to drink.

Many variations are possible. For instance, you could add half a teaspoon of tomato purée (paste), a few drops of lemon juice, a pinch of
dried garlic granules or a sprinkling of freshly ground black pepper.

Miso does contain salt, so beware of making your soup too strong.

What it's good for

Why buy packets of artificial ingredients to make instant soup when you can use natural, healthy ones? Miso originates from Japan. It is made from fermented soybeans, with a flavour similar to yeast extract. It is a good source of minerals and B-vitamins and also contains a little protein. It is said by Oriental health experts to generate and maintain warmth in the body and to combat weakness, poor or upset digestion, proneness to feeling cold, and lowered immunity. It is often used to aid recovery from colds and flu. Miso is very versatile and can be used to flavour soups and stews, and to make stock or broth.

Seaweed is rich in iodine, which is often lacking in terrestrial foods. Iodine is needed to support the health of the thyroid gland and also to prevent excessive oestrogen production by the body.

22. Hungarian mushroom soup

175 g/6 oz button mushrooms, thinly sliced
6 shallots, peeled and cut in quarters lengthwise
600 ml/1 pint/2 cups hot vegetable stock (broth)
1 level tbsp rice flour or wheat flour
2 tbsp butter
2 tbsp sour cream
1 tsp paprika
1 tbsp tomato purée (paste)
Low-sodium salt and freshly ground black pepper

Melt the butter in a saucepan over a medium heat, add the shallots and stir-fry for a few minutes until they soften and begin to brown. Sprinkle the flour over the shallots, and stir it in thoroughly.

Now add the hot stock, and stir briskly until the mixture thickens. Stir in the paprika powder, mushroom slices and the tomato purée. Bring the mixture to a simmer then put a lid on the pan and turn the heat down to simmer very gently for 20 minutes, stirring from time to time.

At the end of the cooking time, remove the pan from the heat. Stir in the sour cream, taste the soup and add a little salt if necessary (you may not need any if you used a stock cube). Season with freshly ground black pepper and serve immediately.

What it's good for

Mushrooms are a good source of chromium, a trace element needed for good blood sugar control and diabetes prevention. They are also rich in B-vitamins, iron, copper and zinc.

Paprika is made from dried sweet peppers which have been ground to a powder. The red colour means it is rich in antioxidant carotenes.

Shallots are a member of the onion family, and have a creamy, sweet flavour. Like garlic and other members of the family, they are rich in sulphur compounds which help to protect us against cancer and also help our bodies to eliminate 'heavy' (toxic) metals such as lead and mercury.

23. Italian tomato and parsley soup

2 x 400 ml/14 fl oz cans Italian chopped plum tomatoes
600 ml/1 pint/2 cups vegetable stock (broth)
1 large handful fresh, flat-leaf parsley, finely chopped
150 ml/5 fl oz/½ cup brown rice, soaked in twice its volume of
    water for at least 1 hour (preferably overnight) then drained
2 sticks celery, finely diced
1 large carrot, finely diced
1 medium onion, finely diced
1 clove garlic, crushed
4 tbsp extra-virgin olive oil
Low-sodium salt and freshly ground black pepper
Parmesan cheese

Gently sweat the onion, garlic, celery and carrot together with the olive oil in a large saucepan over a low heat. When tender, stir in the parsley, chopped tomatoes and their juice, stock and brown rice. Bring to the boil over a high heat, then turn the heat down and simmer gently for 45 minutes, stirring occasionally. Taste the soup and add a little salt if necessary (you may not need any if you used a stock cube). Season with freshly ground black pepper and Parmesan cheese.

Variation

This soup is very good with bite-sized chunks of filleted white fish (such as cod or haddock) added five minutes before the end of the cooking time. The fish is cooked when it is opaque and flakes easily.

What it's good for

Although they are canned, Italian chopped plum tomatoes were picked for this recipe rather than fresh ones because of their natural deep-red colour. This red colour is a pigment known as lycopene, and is a powerful antioxidant. Population studies suggest that people who consume lots of lycopene-rich foods have a lower risk of not only prostate cancer, but also cancer of the cervix, skin, bladder, breast, lung and digestive tract. The redder the tomato, the more lycopene it contains. The tomato is also an excellent source of folic acid, vitamin C and potassium.

24. Potage de Crécy

4 SERVINGS

4 large carrots, cleaned and cut into chunks
8 shallots, peeled and quartered lengthwise
1.2 litres/2 pints/4 cups vegetable stock (broth)
4 tbsp brown rice
2 tbsp butter
1 pinch fresh thyme leaves
Low-sodium salt and freshly ground black pepper
Crème fraîche and fresh chopped parsley to garnish

Place the stock, brown rice and carrot chunks in a saucepan, bring to the boil, cover the pan and simmer for 30 minutes, by which time the ingredients should be tender.

Meanwhile, melt the butter in a frying pan (skillet) over a medium heat and add the shallots. Cook over a low to medium heat until tender. Do not allow the shallots to brown. Once cooked, remove from the heat.

When the carrots and rice have finished cooking, remove the pan from the heat and use a hand blender to whizz the ingredients. Don't worry if the soup does not become completely smooth – it is fine for little pieces of rice to remain visible.

Now stir the shallots and thyme leaves into the saucepan and warm through for a couple of minutes. Taste the soup and add a little salt if necessary (you may not need any if you used a stock cube). Season with freshly ground black pepper and serve with a spoonful of crème fraîche and some fresh chopped parsley.

What it's good for

This is the most delicious carrot dish – a wonderful way to get all the carotene goodness, vitamins and pectin fibre that carrots provide. The butter in this dish actually helps you to absorb beta-carotene, which your body uses to make vitamin A. Beta-carotene cannot be absorbed if there is no oil or fat in the meal.

Thyme has antiseptic properties and is also a carminative, helping to relax the stomach and reduce gas formation. It is also rich in anti-oxidants. Drinking tea made from thyme is said to be a folk cure for alcoholism.

Crème fraîche is nowadays easily found in supermarkets. It is made by heating buttermilk or yoghurt with double cream and then letting it stand until thickened. It keeps for much longer without spoiling, and is ideal for adding to soup as it does not curdle. The flavour of crème fraîche is slightly acidic.

25. Broad bean soup with apple and radish

1 cup fresh (shelled) or frozen broad beans (fava beans)
2 cups boiling water
2 large eating apples, cored and diced*
15 cm/6 inch piece of white mooli radish (daikon), peeled and
    diced†
1 tbsp flax oil
1 tsp fresh sage, finely chopped, or ½ tsp dried sage
Low-sodium salt and freshly ground black pepper
Garnish: a sprig of fresh sage or mint

* Choose a variety with a good flavour such as Cox's

† Long white radishes available in ethnic greengrocers and some supermarkets.

Put the water, apples and radish into a saucepan and bring to the boil. Simmer for 10 minutes, then add the beans and simmer for another five minutes or until tender. Using a hand blender, whizz the soup until smooth, then strain through a sieve into a temporary container. Use a ladle to help you push the soup through the sieve, then discard the remaining pulp of apple and bean skins. Return to the saucepan and stir in the sage. Season with a little salt and freshly ground black pepper. Without allowing it to boil, gently reheat the soup. Before serving, whisk in the flax oil and garnish the soup with a sprig of fresh sage or mint.

What it's good for

This is a lovely light soup, perfect for the summer or as a starter. Beans help control cholesterol, insulin and blood sugar, and prevent constipation. They provide protein and B-vitamins. In Oriental medicine, it is believed that broad beans help to drive off water retention and aid weight-loss. Radishes are said to do a similar job, and also help to break down mucus and to balance the thyroid gland.

Apples make this soup light and delicious. Rich in vitamin C and pectin, but providing only about 50 calories each, they are a great aid to losing weight, especially when cooked and eaten warm, when they are so much more filling. Cooking breaks down tough cellulose in plant foods, allowing better digestion.

Sage is used by medical herbalists to treat menopausal problems. It also has antiseptic and antifungal properties, and can be used as a mouthwash, and is reported to have memory-enhancing effects. In Chinese medicine, sage is thought to help release excess water from the body.

26. Quick and easy cream of tomato soup

4–6 SERVINGS

1 x 500 g/1 lb carton passata*
600 ml/1 pint/2 cups hot water
1 x 400 ml/14 fl oz can Italian chopped tomatoes in juice
2 tbsp dairy or soy cream or crème fraîche
1 tsp dried onion granules
1 tsp dried mixed herbs†
½ tsp dried garlic granules
Low-sodium salt and freshly ground black pepper
Garnish: fresh parsley
Optional: 1 tbsp of shelled pumpkin seeds

* Sieved tomatoes: an Italian ingredient often used to make pasta sauce.

† Rosemary, oregano, marjoram, tarragon, sage, bay leaf, parsley and chives are all good.

Pour the passata, water and chopped tomatoes into a saucepan over a medium heat. Stir in the mixed herbs, onion and garlic granules, and bring to the boil, stirring. Reduce the heat to the lowest setting, stir in the cream and warm through for a minute without boiling. Taste and add a little salt. Stir again, season with freshly ground black pepper and serve garnished with parsley.

If this soup is for someone with an enlarged prostate, you may wish to add pumpkin seeds, which are very helpful for this problem. Dry-roast the shelled seeds in a frying pan over a medium heat for two minutes, then allow to cool and crush in a mortar and pestle. Sprinkle the crushed seeds over the soup before serving.

What it's good for

Ready just as quickly as canned soup, this one tastes so good! The natural deep-red colour of canned Italian tomatoes makes them very healthy. This colour is a natural, nutritious pigment known as lycopene, and is a powerful antioxidant. Population studies suggest that people who consume lots of lycopene-rich foods have a lower risk of not only prostate cancer, but also cancer of the cervix, skin, bladder, breast, lung and digestive tract. The redder the tomato, the more lycopene it contains. The tomato is also a good source of folic acid, vitamin C and potassium. And it's okay to indulge in some fresh cream from time to time. After all, dairy cream is a source of retinol (real vitamin A) and vitamin D, which are not found in most other foods.

27. Quick and easy cream of vegetable soup

4 SERVINGS

3 cups frozen, diced mixed vegetables*

1.2 litres/2 pints/4 cups boiling water

1 medium potato, cut into quarters lengthwise then thinly sliced

1 large onion, chopped

1 large tomato, skinned and diced†

2 tbsp olive oil

2 tbsp dairy or soy cream or crème fraîche

2 tsp dried or 2 tbsp fresh or frozen parsley

1 chicken or vegetable stock cube

Low-sodium salt and freshly ground black pepper

* Most combinations work well but the vegetables need to be in small pieces. A good combination is peas, carrots, sweetcorn kernels, peppers and green beans.

† To skin tomatoes, leave them in a bowl of boiling water for 60 seconds, then drain and rinse with cold water. Use a sharp knife to remove the peel, which should come off easily.

Place the stock cube in a cup and fill with boiling water. Stir to dissolve. Place the stock, the rest of the hot water, mixed vegetables, potato and onion in a large saucepan over a medium heat and stir well together. Put a lid on the pan, bring it to the boil then turn down the heat to the lowest setting and leave for 15 minutes or until the vegetables are tender.

Add the olive oil, then, using a hand blender, whizz the contents of the pan for about 10 seconds, until you have a half-smooth, half-chunky consistency. Stir in the diced tomato, parsley and cream, then taste the soup and add a little salt if necessary. Serve seasoned with freshly ground black pepper.

Variations

A few cooked beans or some cooked diced ham can also be added after blending. Heat through gently for two minutes before serving.

28. Roasted Mediterranean vegetable soup

4 SERVINGS

2 large courgettes (zucchini), cut into chunks

1 aubergine (eggplant), cut into chunks

1 sweet green (bell) pepper, cut in half, stalks and seeds removed

1 sweet yellow (bell) pepper, cut in half, stalks and seeds removed

2 large tomatoes, skins scored around the waist

2 tbsp tomato purée (paste) dissolved in 600 ml/1 pint/2 cups hot water

1 large onion, quartered

1 head of garlic, separated into cloves and peeled

Sprigs of fresh herbs (rosemary, marjoram, sage and/or thyme are all good)

Extra-virgin olive oil

Low-sodium salt and freshly ground black pepper

Garnish: grated cheese, Greek yoghurt and black olive halves

Preheat the oven to 190°C/375°F/Gas Mark 5.

Drizzle or spray a large roasting tray with olive oil, then arrange the vegetable pieces in a single layer. Lightly crush the garlic cloves under the flat of a knife. Scatter the garlic cloves among the vegetables, then drizzle or spray the vegetables liberally with olive oil, and scatter the sprigs of fresh herbs over the top. Place the tray on the top rung of the preheated oven and roast for 45 minutes or until the vegetables are tender, the onions are browning and the pepper skins are beginning to blacken. Halfway through the cooking time, drizzle/spray the vegetables with more olive oil.

When the vegetables are cooked, remove the tray from the oven. Remove and discard the herb sprigs. Using a spatula, lift the peppers out of the tray and wrap them in a plastic bag or some clingfilm for five minutes. Remove the skins from the tomatoes and cut the tomatoes into chunks. Put half the tomato chunks, garlic and other vegetable pieces into a food processor and the other half in a saucepan. Put half a cup of water into the empty roasting tray and deglaze the pan with a spatula by scraping off all the flavour-rich remains of the vegetables. Pour the resulting deglaze liquid into the saucepan.

Now remove the peppers from the plastic, slip off their skins and cut the flesh into strips. Put half the peppers into the food processor and the other half into the saucepan.

Switch on the processor and process the vegetables to a rough purée. Add the purée to the saucepan and stir in the tomato-flavoured water. Warm the soup over a medium heat until it just begins to bubble. Taste the soup and add a little salt if necessary. Season with freshly ground black pepper. Serve on wide, shallow stew plates, sprinkled with grated cheese and topped with black olive halves and a spoonful of Greek yoghurt.

What it's good for

This soup requires a little extra preparation, but the result is well worth it. Roasting vegetables intensifies their flavours, and this soup becomes a rich and satisfying meal. The healthy reputation of the Mediterranean diet owes much to its vegetables and olive oil. These ingredients form part of a popular dish known as ratatouille, which originates from the south of France.

29. Russian lemon soup

1 lemon

4 tbsp brown rice*

4 cups chicken stock (broth)

1 tbsp fresh parsley, finely chopped

2 tbsp dairy or soy cream

Low-sodium salt and freshly ground black pepper

* You could also use leftover cooked rice. Just double the quantity and reduce the cooking time of the soup to 15 minutes.

Put the stock and rice in a saucepan and bring to the boil. Turn down the heat to the lowest setting, place a lid on the pan and simmer gently for 35 minutes. Meanwhile, grate 1 teaspoon of zest off the lemon and reserve to one side. Juice the rest of the lemon.

At the end of the cooking time, stir in the cream, parsley, lemon juice and zest. Taste the soup and add a little salt if necessary (you may not need any if you used a stock cube). Season with freshly ground black pepper before serving.

Variation

To increase the protein content (and obtain the benefits of soy foods), omit the cream and instead stir in some diced tofu.

What it's good for

Lemon juice is rich in vitamin C and the zest is rich in flavonoids. By keeping the walls of small blood vessels strong, flavonoids are needed to prevent problems with the microcirculation, such as Alzheimer's disease, varicose veins and eyesight and ear problems. Parsley is rich in vitamin C and also contains coumarin, which helps your immune system to break down protein particles that have leaked into your tissue spaces, and lie there attracting water retention. Brown rice is rich in B-vitamins and also provides a little protein.

30. South Indian spicy sambhar soup

2 cups mixed vegetables*, cut into 1 cm/½ inch pieces

1 large tomato, chopped

2 long, thin chilli peppers

2 tbsp cooked red lentils[†]

2 tbsp olive oil

1 level tbsp mango powder[§]

Boiling water

FLAVOURINGS

A few dried curry leaves

1 tbsp chopped fresh coriander

1 tsp turmeric

½ tsp each of whole spices: black mustard, fenugreek and cumin
seeds

½ tsp each of ground spices: cinnamon, coriander, asafetida, black
pepper, cayenne pepper

Low-sodium salt

* It is fine to use frozen chopped mixed vegetables if you wish. Do not allow them
to defrost before cooking.

† To cook red lentils, simmer in 2¼ times their volume of water plus a tablespoon of
oil in a covered pan for 25 minutes, stirring from time to time. Remove from the heat
and beat with a wooden spoon to form a purée. If you make extra you can freeze
the remainder to make other soups.

§ Available from Asian shops. If you cannot get it, use a tablespoon of tomato purée
(paste) instead.

Using a sharp fork, prick the chillies all the way down their length, leaving them whole. This will release their flavour while keeping them whole so that you can avoid eating them if you wish.

Measure out the whole spices into a small bowl. Measure out the turmeric and other ground spices into a separate small bowl.

Using a large saucepan with a heavy base, heat the oil and the whole spices together. When the mustard seeds begin to pop, add the chilli peppers and all the vegetables except the tomato. Stir-fry for two minutes.

Now stir in the ground spices and turmeric. Add the curry leaves, mango powder (or tomato purée), chopped tomato and just enough hot water to cover the ingredients. Place a lid on the pan, bring to a gentle simmer, and cook for 35 minutes.

Stir in the cooked lentils and chopped fresh coriander and simmer for five more minutes. Taste the soup and add a little salt if necessary. Sambhar is traditionally a fiery dish. If you find it too spicy, cut down on the cayenne pepper or add it at the end to gauge how much you prefer.

What it's good for

Sambhar is a staple dish in south India. It is eaten as a soup or with rice. Always fiery, sambhar owes its heat to the chilli (cayenne) pepper, which has great health benefits, especially for the circulation. This is just the dish to eat if you feel a cold coming on. Chillies also stimulate the digestion and help prevent flatulence.

31. Vichyssoise

3 large leeks
2 medium potatoes, peeled and diced
600 ml/1 pint/2 cups vegetable stock (broth)
3 tbsp dairy or soy cream
2 tbsp butter
Low-sodium salt and freshly ground black pepper
Garnish: chopped fresh chives

Trim the ends off the leeks, then cut them in half lengthwise and chop into 2.5 cm/1 inch lengths. Place in a sink of cold water, rub together with your hands to remove any grit, then drain with a colander.

Place the leeks in a large saucepan over a medium heat and sweat gently in the butter until beginning to soften. Now add the potatoes and stir in the stock. Bring to the boil, cover the pan and simmer gently for 30 minutes. Remove from the heat.

Using a hand blender, whizz the contents of the pan until completely smooth, then stir in the cream. Taste the soup and add a little salt if necessary (you may not need any if you used a stock cube). Serve seasoned with freshly ground black pepper and garnished with chopped chives.

Variation

This soup is also delicious with cooked or canned butterbeans (lima beans) added after you have whizzed the ingredients. After adding them, just return the soup to the heat for a minute or two to heat through, and then stir in the cream. This increases the protein content of this soup, and you could also sprinkle on some cheese.

What it's good for

Leeks belong to the onion family and have similar health benefits. Rich in sulphur compounds, they help to protect us against cancer and also help our bodies to eliminate 'heavy' (toxic) metals such as lead and mercury.

32. Watercress soup

225 g/8 oz/4 cups fresh watercress, finely chopped*
600 ml/1 pint/2 cups vegetable stock (broth)
2 medium potatoes, diced
1 large onion, diced
2 tbsp dairy or soy cream
Low-sodium salt and freshly ground black pepper

* This soup is also good for using up any salad leaves, such as lettuce or rocket, which are no longer fresh.

Put the watercress, stock, diced potatoes and chopped onion in a saucepan and bring to the boil. Simmer for 25 minutes or until the ingredients are tender. Remove from the heat and whizz with a hand blender. Taste the soup and add a little salt if necessary (you may not need any if you used a stock cube). Just before serving, stir in the cream and season with black pepper.

What it's good for

Watercress is a leafy green vegetable and so is rich in antioxidants such as carotenes and vitamin C, folic acid and the minerals calcium and magnesium. It is related to the cabbage and broccoli family of vegetables, which is renowned for helping to prevent cancer. Recent research has in fact shown that watercress has good anti-cancer properties, especially for smokers.

SUBSTANTIAL SOUPS
(ONE-POT MEALS)

33. Broccoli cream soup with Stilton cheese

2–4 SERVINGS

1 litre/1¾ pints/3½ cups soy milk
1 medium head of broccoli
55 g/2 oz Stilton cheese, crumbled
2 tbsp butter
1 slightly rounded tbsp rice flour or wheat flour
Low-sodium salt and freshly ground black pepper

Using a sharp knife or peeler, peel the thick stem of the broccoli and then cut if off and chop roughly. Cut the broccoli head into florets and then cut these into bite-sized pieces.

Place all the broccoli pieces in a saucepan with the milk and bring to the boil. Simmer gently for 10 minutes or until the broccoli is tender.

Using a sieve or colander, strain the milk into a temporary container. Put the broccoli to one side and keep warm.

Clean the saucepan thoroughly, then replace it over a low heat and make a white sauce. To do this, melt the butter then add the flour and stir with a wooden spoon until you obtain a paste. Stir this paste briskly for 1–2 minutes. Now pour in the hot milk, and immediately whisk it to prevent lumps from forming. Bring the mixture to the boil, then simmer for five minutes until it thickens, stirring all the time to prevent it sticking.

Stir half the broccoli pieces into the sauce and use a hand blender to whizz the mixture until smooth. (The blender will also get rid of any lumps which may have developed in the sauce.)

Now stir in the crumbled Stilton cheese and keep stirring until it has melted. Taste the soup and add a little salt if necessary (the cheese may already contain salt). Gently fold in the cooked broccoli and season with freshly ground black pepper before serving.

What it's good for

Broccoli is now well-known for its anti-cancer properties. This is because it contains ingredients that help your liver break down waste products. These wastes include residues of hormones such as oestrogen which the body no longer requires. Because of this, broccoli is very useful for helping to prevent female health problems such as cysts and endometriosis, which are related to excessively high oestrogen levels.

The soy milk in this recipe also helps to control oestrogen, and has benefits for prostate health and preventing high cholesterol too. Soy milk is not as rich in calcium and protein as cow's milk, but broccoli and cheese help to make up for this as they are both excellent sources of calcium, and cheese is a good source of protein.

34. Brown lentil soup with roasted sweet peppers and apricots

2 SERVINGS

150 ml/5 fl oz/½ cup brown lentils, measured in a measuring jug
850 ml/1½ pints/3 cups boiling water
1 red and one green sweet (bell) pepper
6 fresh or dried apricots, with stones removed, roughly chopped*
1 tbsp brown rice miso
Low-sodium salt and freshly ground black pepper
Garnish: dairy or soy yoghurt

* Unsulphured apricots are dark-brown and sweet. Dried apricots treated with preservatives are orange in colour and have a tangy flavour. As the preservative can irritate your digestive system, these are best scrubbed before use.

Put the peppers under the grill (broiler) and cook until the skins begin to blacken. Keep turning them over so that they blacken evenly on all sides.

Place the blackened peppers in a plastic bag and leave to cool. Meanwhile put the lentils and water in a saucepan, bring to the boil, cover and simmer for 30 minutes or until tender. Stir in the miso and keep stirring until it has dissolved. Using a hand blender, whizz the lentils for a few seconds until the soup begins to thicken but there are still plenty of whole lentils. Then add the apricots and return to the heat. Bring back to the boil and simmer for another 10 minutes.

Remove the peppers from the plastic bag and peel off the skin, which should come away easily. Cut the peppers into thin strips and stir them into the soup. Taste the soup and add a little salt if necessary (miso already contains salt). Heat through, season with freshly ground black pepper and decorate with a swirl of yoghurt before serving.

What it's good for

Lentils are a good source of vegetarian protein and soluble fibre, plus iron, zinc and B-vitamins. The iron from plant foods such as lentils is not well absorbed unless the meal also contains a good source of vitamin C. In this soup the vitamin C is provided by the peppers, and these will help you to absorb iron from the lentils. Drinking a glass of orange juice with this soup will also help you absorb this iron.

Dried fruit (such as apricots) is rich in potassium and many other minerals. However, it does not contain any vitamin C.

Miso is a Japanese flavouring used to make soup. Rich in B-vitamins and made from fermented soybeans, it is considered one of Japan's premier health foods.

35. Brussels butterbean bisque

4 SERVINGS

225 g/8 oz Brussels sprouts, trimmed and cut in quarters lengthwise
1.2 litres/2 pints/4 cups vegetable stock (broth)*
1 x 400 g/14 oz can butterbeans (lima beans), rinsed and drained†
6 shallots, peeled and cut in quarters lengthwise
Olive oil
Low-sodium salt and freshly ground black pepper

* During the four-day detox, avoid using salted stock and try not to add salt to this soup.

† Or use a cup of home-cooked beans (see page 272)

Place the butterbeans and stock in a saucepan over a medium heat. Bring to the boil and simmer for 10 minutes. Whizz with a hand blender until smooth.

Meanwhile, put 2 tablespoons of olive oil and 2 tablespoons of water in a wide frying pan (skillet) over a medium heat. Place the Brussels sprouts in the pan in a single layer, and cover the pan tightly. Allow the sprouts to cook for a few minutes, shaking the pan occasionally until the water has evaporated and the sprouts are beginning to soften and brown a little.

Using a slotted spoon, transfer the sprouts and their oil to the saucepan of blended beans. Add another 2 tablespoons of olive oil and 2 tablespoons of water to the frying pan, and cook the shallots in the same way as you cooked the sprouts. When this is done, add the shallots and their oil to the saucepan with the other ingredients.

Now bring the saucepan to simmering point and simmer very gently for 15 minutes, stirring occasionally. Taste the soup and add a little salt if necessary (you may not need any if you used a stock cube). Season with freshly ground black pepper before serving.

What it's good for

Thanks to the butterbeans, this soup tastes as if it has been made with lavish amounts of cream, yet is actually quite low in fat. Butterbeans are a good source of fibre, vegetarian protein, B-vitamins, zinc and molybdenum (a trace element needed for detoxification).

Brussels sprouts belong to the cabbage and broccoli family of vegetables and are one of its most powerful members contributing to the prevention of breast cancer.

36. Butternut bisque
with Cajun-style red mullet

1 small butternut squash

1.2 litres/2 pints/4 cups soy milk

4 red mullet fillets

1 large onion, finely chopped

2 tbsp olive oil

4 tbsp groundnut oil

2 tbsp Cajun spice mix*

Freshly ground black pepper

Alfalfa sprouts to garnish†

* You can buy this in supermarkets, or grind the following ingredients together with a mortar and pestle: 2 tsp onion powder, 2 tsp garlic powder, 2 tsp dried thyme or oregano, 1 tsp cayenne pepper, 1 tsp ground black pepper

† You can buy alfalfa sprouts from health-food stores, or make your own (see page 273)

Preheat the oven to 190°C/375°F/Gas Mark 5.

Cut the squash in half lengthways, and remove the seeds with a spoon. Lay the squash pieces cut side down on a greased baking tray and bake in the preheated oven for 30 minutes or until tender.

Meanwhile, sweat the onion in the olive oil in a small covered pan over a low heat until soft. Heat the soy milk in a large saucepan.

When the squash is tender, scoop the flesh out of the skin and add half to the pan of hot soy milk, together with the chopped onion. Using a hand blender, whizz the ingredients until smooth. Gradually whizz in the rest of the squash. (Don't add it all if you find the soup is becoming too thick.) Keep the pan on a very low heat while you prepare the fish.

Spread the Cajun spice mix out on a plate. Dry the fish fillets with absorbent kitchen paper, then press both sides firmly into the powder until they are thickly coated.

Heat the groundnut oil in a frying pan (skillet) over a high heat. When the oil is very hot, turn the heat down to medium, add the fish fillets, flesh side down, and cook for one minute. Turn over and cook the other side for half a minute (or until the fish is cooked through), pressing down with a spatula to prevent the fillets from curling up. Drain briefly on kitchen paper.

Ladle the soup into shallow bowls, season with freshly ground black pepper, then place a fish fillet in the centre of each. Garnish with alfalfa sprouts.

The flavour of this soup is sweet, and it is best left unsalted. If you do add salt, do so very carefully, as more than a very tiny pinch will spoil the soup.

Variations

Use mackerel fillets instead of red mullet. For a delicious vegetarian version, sprinkle this soup with a handful of Emmenthal cheese instead of adding fish.

What it's good for

Like carrots and orange-flesh sweet potatoes, butternut squash is rich in cancer-preventing carotenes. Soy milk forms a useful part of your diet if you suffer from a high oestrogen or enlarged prostate problem. Soy products are also recommended by the medical establishment to help control cholesterol levels. The best thing about this soup is that it tastes like something made with lavish amounts of cream, yet it is quite low in calories.

The Cajun spices warm your circulation and help to fight water retention. Fish is of course a great source of protein, zinc, iodine, selenium and other minerals, which are lacking nowadays in plant foods in many parts of the world.

37. Carrot, chicken and sweetcorn spicy chowder

4 SERVINGS

1.2 litres/2 pints/4 cups water

Half an organic chicken, jointed*

1 cup fresh or frozen sweetcorn kernels

1 large carrot, diced small

1 large onion, diced

1 large potato, diced

4 tbsp dairy or soy cream

2 tbsp brown rice

1 clove garlic, crushed

1 tsp fresh tarragon, chopped

½ tsp dried chilli flakes

Low-sodium salt

Put the water, chicken pieces, onion, garlic, rice and potato in a saucepan, bring to the boil and simmer for 45 minutes or until all the chicken pieces are cooked through. Using a fork or slotted spoon, remove the chicken pieces and put to one side while the next set of ingredients is cooking. Using a hand blender, whizz the remaining contents of the pan until no more pieces of potato are visible.

Now stir the chilli flakes, diced carrot, corn kernels and tarragon into the pan, and simmer for another 15 minutes until the vegetables are tender. Just before serving, remove the bones and skin from the chicken and cut the flesh into small pieces. Add these to the soup and stir in the cream. Taste the soup and add a little salt if necessary. Heat through gently (without boiling) for two minutes before serving.

What it's good for

Chicken is a good source of protein, and is low in animal fat. It provides B-vitamins, zinc and other nutrients needed by your immune system. Sweetcorn also provides a little protein, as well as starch and essential polyunsaturated oils. Its deep-yellow colour is due to carotenes, which have cancer-prevention properties.

Tarragon has a slightly aniseed flavour and goes particularly well with chicken. Fresh tarragon has much more flavour than dried. Tea made from tarragon is said to help relieve flatulence, promote sleep and to have a mild diuretic action which helps the body flush out toxins produced by eating too much protein.

38. Chinese egg and spring onion soup

2 SERVINGS

2 cups vegetable stock (broth)
4 spring onions (scallions), thinly sliced
1 tsp grated fresh ginger
1 tbsp fresh chopped parsley
1 level tbsp cornflour (cornstarch)
1 egg
Low-sodium salt and white pepper

Place the stock, grated ginger, spring onions and chopped parsley in a saucepan over a medium heat. Meanwhile, using a small bowl, mix the cornflour into a smooth paste with 2 tablespoons of water. Whisk the egg.

When the stock boils, turn down the heat to its lowest setting. Slowly stir in the cornflour paste, and keep stirring until the soup thickens.

Pour the egg into the soup in a thin stream, while gently stirring the soup in a clockwise direction (anticlockwise if you are left-handed). Remove the pan from the heat, taste the soup and season with salt (if necessary) and white pepper. If you used a stock cube, the soup may not need any salt.

Variations

Chinese restaurants use this method to make the well-known chicken and sweetcorn soup. You too can make this simply by adding sweetcorn kernels and cooked shredded chicken to the stock.

What it's good for

This is a light soup, good for those recovering from illness, when extra protein is needed. Egg is a good source of protein and is rather under-used in soups. Egg yolk also provides nutrients such as zinc and a small amount of vitamins A, D and E. Although egg yolks contain cholesterol, it is the cholesterol made within the body as a result of eating too little fibre and too much sugar and animal fat which mostly clogs arteries. In fact, the American Heart Association approves an intake of up to four eggs a week.

39. Chinese hot and sour soup

1.2 litres/2 pints/4 cups hot chicken stock (broth)

450 g/1 lb pack frozen Chinese or Thai stir-fry vegetables

110 g/4 oz shiitake mushrooms (caps only), sliced*

110 g/4 oz bean curd or tofu, drained and cut into 1 cm/½ inch cubes

2 eggs, beaten

2 cloves garlic, crushed

2 tbsp dark soy sauce

1 level dessertspoon psyllium husks

2 tbsp apple cider vinegar

2 tsp chilli paste

1 tsp sesame oil

Garnish: 2 spring onions (scallions), thinly sliced

* If you can get Chinese 'black fungus' mushrooms and straw mushrooms (Chinese supermarkets sell them dried or in cans), you can use a mixture of these instead. Black fungus needs to be soaked in warm water for 10 minutes and then rinsed before use.

Put the hot stock in a saucepan, sprinkle in the psyllium husks and quickly whisk (using a balloon whisk) to incorporate them. Now add the frozen vegetables and bring to the boil. Add the soy sauce, vinegar, garlic, mushrooms and chilli paste. Simmer (stirring occasionally) for 15 minutes or until the vegetables are just tender. Now add the bean curd and heat through for a minute.

Pour the eggs into the soup in a thin stream while you stir it in a clockwise direction (anticlockwise if you are left-handed). Allow to stand for half a minute, then add the sesame oil and serve the soup with a garnish of chopped spring onions. This soup should not need any salt as soy sauce is quite salty.

What it's good for

In Oriental medicine, it is considered important that every meal should balance the five main flavours: sweet, salty, sour, bitter and pungent. This is the reason for combining several flavours in this soup. Mushrooms and many vegetables such as cabbage and carrots are classed as sweet, while onions, garlic and spices are classed as pungent.

Despite their unappealing name, black fungus mushrooms have a reputation in Chinese herbal medicine for increasing the fluidity of the blood and improving the circulation. They are given to patients suffering from arteriosclerosis, and help to prevent strokes and heart attacks.

Psyllium husks are used here as a thickener instead of the more traditional cornflour or cornstarch. Consisting of soluble fibre, they are perfect for helping to prevent constipation, and also for bowel health in general. By delaying the absorption of carbohydrates, soluble fibre also helps to control insulin levels.

40. Cream of cauliflower soup

2-4 SERVINGS

1 cauliflower

1 x 400 g/14 oz can butterbeans (lima beans), rinsed and drained*

600 ml/1 pint/2 cups hot vegetable or chicken stock (broth)†

2 tbsp olive oil

Freshly grated nutmeg

Low-sodium salt and freshly ground black pepper

Boiling water

To garnish: alfalfa sprouts

* Or use a cup of home-cooked beans (see page 272).

† During the four-day detox, avoid using salted stock and try not to add salt to this soup.

Chop the cauliflower into small pieces. Put the stock in a saucepan and add the cauliflower and butterbeans. Add enough boiling water just to cover the ingredients. Bring to the boil and simmer for about 15 minutes or until the cauliflower is tender. Remove from the heat and add the olive oil to the pan. Using a hand blender, whizz the soup until completely smooth, then pass through a sieve to remove any remaining pieces of bean skin. Return the soup to the pan and heat through gently without boiling. Taste the soup and add a little salt if necessary (you may not need any if you used a stock cube). Season with freshly grated nutmeg and freshly ground black pepper, and serve garnished with alfalfa sprouts.

Variations

This soup can also be cooked with soy milk instead of stock.

What it's good for

As a white vegetable, cauliflower does not have all the antioxidant goodness of yellow, green and red vegetables. Nevertheless it is a member of the cabbage family, and so contains substances that help your liver process toxins and hormonal wastes such as used oestrogen. Adding butterbeans not only gives this soup a lovely creamy consistency, but also increases its protein content.

41. Cream of mushroom soup with shiitake

3–4 SERVINGS

225 g/8 oz fresh open-cap mushrooms, roughly chopped
1 medium onion, roughly chopped
1 litre/1¾ pints/3½ cups soy milk
4 shiitake mushrooms (caps only), thinly sliced
1 rounded tbsp brown rice miso
1 slightly rounded tbsp rice flour or wheat flour
1 tbsp fresh parsley, finely chopped
Olive oil
2 tbsp soy cream (optional)
Low-sodium salt and freshly ground black pepper

Heat the soy milk to just below boiling point in a saucepan. Remove from the heat.

Meanwhile, heat 2 tbsp olive oil in a large saucepan over a medium heat and sweat the chopped onion for a few minutes until translucent. Add the chopped open-cap mushrooms, turning up the heat so that their juices will not collect in the pan. Stir-fry briskly for about three minutes. Sprinkle the flour over the mushrooms and stir it in thoroughly.

Now add about a cupful of the hot soy milk, and stir briskly until the mixture thickens. Stir in the rest of the hot soy milk. Stir in the miso and keep stirring until it has dissolved. Bring the mixture to simmering point then turn the heat down and simmer very gently for 20 minutes, stirring from time to time.

While this is happening, heat 1 tbsp olive oil in a small frying pan (skillet) and stir-fry the shiitake mushroom slices over a medium heat for a minute or two until golden but not crisp. Remove from the heat, drain with a slotted spoon and reserve to one side.

When the soup has reached the end of its 20 minutes cooking time, remove it from the heat. Using a hand blender, whizz the soup in the pan until you achieve the consistency you want. Stir in the soy cream if using, the shiitake mushroom slices and chopped parsley. Taste the soup and add a little salt if necessary (miso already contains salt). Before serving, season with freshly ground black pepper.

Variation

If you wish to increase the calcium and protein content of this soup, add a tablespoon of cottage cheese just before serving.

What it's good for

The main benefit of mushrooms is their vitamin and mineral content. They are rich in B-vitamins, iron, copper, zinc and chromium. Shiitake mushrooms contain lentinan, a substance with anti-cancer properties. They are frequently recommended by doctors in Japan.

You could use cow's milk to make this soup but I have chosen soy milk. This is not so rich in calcium but has many health benefits, including helping to control cholesterol and oestrogen levels and prevent prostate problems.

42. German marrowfat pea soup with sausage

225 g/8 oz/1 cup dried marrowfat peas
110 g/4 oz/firm, low-fat soup sausage such as cabanos, cut into
    bite-sized chunks*
2 medium potatoes, diced
3 medium carrots, cut into chunks
1 large onion or 1 leek, cut into chunks
1 tbsp brown rice miso (or you could use a stock cube)
Low-sodium salt and freshly ground black pepper
Boiling water

SPECIAL EQUIPMENT
A pressure cooker

* If in doubt, ask in a delicatessen about suitable products

Pour at least four times their volume of boiling water over the peas, allowing them plenty of room to swell. Leave to soak overnight. If using a leek, cut in half lengthways and then into chunks. Wash thoroughly to remove any grit.

Discard the peas' soaking water, then put the peas in a pressure cooker and cover them with 2.5 cm/1 inch of boiling water. Bring up to full steam, then cook for 10 minutes. Plunge the pressure cooker into a sink of cold water to prevent further cooking and reduce the pressure enough to allow you to open the lid. The peas should be very soft and tender, and some of them mushy. If you don't get this consistency, replace the lid and pressure-cook them again for a few minutes.

Pour the peas and their liquid into an ordinary large saucepan. Stir in the miso or stock cube, ensuring it dissolves completely, followed by the vegetables and sausage pieces. Pour in just enough water to barely cover the ingredients, stir well, then bring back to the boil and simmer over a low heat for one hour, stirring occasionally. If the soup liquid looks a little thin, squash some of the peas with the back of a spoon and stir again.

Taste the soup and add a little salt if necessary (miso and most stock cubes already contain salt). Season with freshly ground black pepper and serve in large shallow stew plates.

Variations

In Germany, all types of vegetables are thrown into this soup and it is good for using up leftovers. You can also cook it with yellow split peas instead of marrowfat peas, or, instead of sausage, add some lean chunks of cooked ham just before the end of the cooking time.

What it's good for

Like beans, marrowfat peas are rich in protein, minerals and B-vitamins, and this dish makes a substantial and highly nutritious meal. Sausages are included because it is traditional to cook this dish with them. Some types are not particularly fatty and a little goes a long way. But do remember that sausages and ham contain preservatives and often quite a lot of salt. Carrots are a rich source of the antioxidant beta-carotene.

It is well worth buying some brown rice miso from your local health-food store. This is a Japanese health food and is much more nutritious than the average stock cube. It contains nothing artificial, and can also be made into a soup in its own right, just by adding hot water.

43. Hungarian minestrone with shallots and brown beans

4 SERVINGS

1 x 400 g/14 oz can of borlotti beans, drained and rinsed*

1 litre/1¾ pints/3½ cups fresh tomato juice from
    a carton

110 g/4 oz shallots, peeled and quartered

2 handfuls dried macaroni

2 sticks celery, finely chopped

2 tomatoes, skinned and chopped†

4 cloves garlic, chopped

Olive oil

1 rounded tsp rice flour or wheat flour

1 tbsp sweet ground paprika

1 tbsp fresh parsley, chopped

Low-sodium salt and freshly ground black pepper

Garnish: sour cream and fresh chopped chives

* If you cannot get these, use pinto or kidney beans instead.

† To skin tomatoes, leave them in a bowl of boiling water for 60 seconds, then drain and rinse with cold water. Use a sharp knife to remove the peel, which should come off easily.

Using a large saucepan with a heavy base, gently fry the shallots, celery and garlic in 2 tbsp olive oil until the shallots begin to soften. Sprinkle the flour over the ingredients, and stir-fry for a few moments until the flour is absorbed. Now add about a cupful of the tomato juice, and stir briskly until the mixture thickens. Stir in the paprika powder followed by the remainder of the tomato juice, and the beans. Bring to the boil then simmer gently for 45 minutes, stirring occasionally.

Meanwhile, cook the macaroni until 'al dente', according to the directions on the packet. Drain, rinse with cold water and drain again. Place the macaroni in a bowl and stir in a tablespoon of olive oil to keep it from sticking together.

Five minutes before the end of the cooking time, stir in the cooked macaroni, chopped tomatoes and parsley. Taste the soup and add a little salt if necessary. Serve the minestrone with a spoonful of sour cream and some fresh chopped chives.

What it's good for

Beans are a good source of vegetarian protein, as well as iron, zinc and B-vitamins. The vitamin C provided by the fresh tomatoes and parsley will help you absorb the iron from the beans.

Shallots are a member of the onion and garlic family, and have similar benefits, such as antihistamine and antiviral effects. Like beans, they are a good source of soluble fibre, which helps to fight high cholesterol.

44. Japanese buckwheat noodle soup

4 SERVINGS

225 g/8 oz Japanese soba (buckwheat) noodles*

600 ml/1 pint/2 cups vegetable or mushroom stock (broth)

110 g/4 oz/1 cup shiitake mushrooms[†], caps only, thinly sliced

2 spring onions (scallions or green onions), thinly sliced

1 sweet red (bell) pepper, cut into thin strips

A few shreds of dried seaweed (kombu or wakame are traditionally used)*

4 large green cabbage leaves (thick veins removed), cut into wide strips

225 g/8 oz firm tofu, drained and cut into 1 cm/½ inch cubes[§]

1 generous thumb-sized piece of fresh ginger, peeled and chopped into tiny matchsticks

1 medium carrot, cut into 3 segments then thinly sliced lengthwise

12 cm/5 inch piece of white mooli radish (daikon), peeled and cut into matchsticks

4 tbsp tamari sauce*

Boiling water

*Available from health-food stores and macrobiotic suppliers. Tamrai is a high-quality gluten-free soy sauce.

[†] If unavailable you can use ordinary white mushrooms instead.

[§] Use a brand with a chewy texture, such as Cauldron. Avoid silken tofu for this recipe.

Build the soup up in layers in a large saucepan. First add the strips of mushroom, then the onions, pepper and seaweed, followed by the cabbage leaves, tofu, ginger, carrot and radish. Pour the mushroom stock and tamari sauce into the pan, plus just enough boiling water to almost cover the ingredients. Bring to the boil over a medium heat and simmer very gently for 45 minutes. Keep the soup warm while you prepare the noodles.

Cook the noodles according to the packet directions, then drain and place in a serving bowl. Ladle the soup over them and serve immediately. This soup should not need any salt because tamari sauce is already quite salty.

What it's good for

Shiitake mushrooms are a traditional health food in Japan, and are being intensely studied by scientists for their antiviral and anti-cancer properties. They have an active ingredient known as lentinan, which works by helping the body's immune system to eliminate tumours. Like the tofu in this recipe, shiitake mushrooms are high in protein. If you can find maitake mushrooms, you could use these instead. Maitake means 'dancing for joy'. It is good for blood sugar regulation, insulin resistance and pre-diabetic states. Like shiitake, it is an approved medicine in Japan, used together with radio- and chemotherapy in cancer therapy.

As a natural soy food with little processing, tofu has many health benefits, including significant cholesterol-lowering properties and as an aid to preventing breast and prostate cancers.

Seaweed is rich in iodine, which is often in short supply and is needed to maintain an efficient metabolism. A diet too low in iodine can also cause women to produce too much oestrogen.

Buckwheat is a good source of B-vitamins and the mineral molybdenum, which is needed by liver enzymes. Despite its name, it is not related to the wheat family, and noodles made from 100 per cent buckwheat are gluten-free.

45. Lemon dal soup

3 types of yellow lentils: half a cup each of channa dal, toor dal,
   moong dal*
6 cups boiling water
1 medium onion, cut in half lengthwise then thinly sliced
1 unwaxed lemon
1 handful fresh coriander, chopped
6 cloves garlic, roughly chopped
4 small chillies
3 tbsp vegetable oil
Low-sodium salt

SPICES AND FLAVOURINGS
3 curry leaves
1 tsp black mustard seeds
1 tsp turmeric
1 tsp cumin seeds
1 pinch asafetida

Garnish: fresh coriander leaves or sprouted green or brown lentils
   (see page 273)

* These are available from Asian shops and are considered the best combination for
making dal. If you prefer, you could use just one variety.

Pick over the dal, looking for any small stones to remove. Place the dal, water, turmeric and 1 tbsp of oil in a large saucepan, stir and bring to the boil. Simmer uncovered for 40 minutes, stirring occasionally and skimming off any scum which rises to the surface. Check the consistency and add a little boiling water if the soup is too thick.

Meanwhile, pare about a quarter of the zest off the lemon and cut it into long, thin shreds. (Alternatively use a lemon zester tool which is designed to make strands.) Cut the lemon in half. Extract the juice from one half and slice the peel off the other half by cutting downwards with a sharp knife. Cut the lemon flesh into small chunks. Reserve all these items.

Prick the chillies all over with a fork so that they can be left whole while still releasing some of their heat. Warm the remaining oil over a medium heat in a stir-fry pan, and add the mustard seeds. When they start to pop, stir in the cumin seeds, followed by the asafetida and curry leaves. Quickly stir in the sliced onion, chillies and garlic, and stir-fry for a few minutes until the onion has softened and is beginning to brown.

At the end of the cooking time, stir the onion mixture, chopped coriander and lemon pieces, juice and zest into the dal, and simmer for another two minutes. Check the seasoning and add a little salt. Serve the dal garnished with fresh coriander leaves or sprouted lentils (see page 273). Unless you like eating whole chillies, remove them before eating. They are mainly for decoration!

What it's good for

This is a meal loaded with power foods. Lentils (dal) are a good source of fibre, iron and B-vitamins. The lemon in this recipe helps you to absorb the iron, which is not well absorbed from plant foods unless you consume some vitamin C at the same time.

Turmeric is a power food for your liver, helping to protect it from toxins and aiding its function. In India, it is considered an excellent arthritis remedy. (The yellow colour is due to the presence of curcumin, one of the most powerful antioxidants in nature.)

Like garlic, ginger and chillies, black mustard seeds are classified in Oriental medicine as a 'pungent' food, which means they help to support the Yang energy that stimulates the metabolism and drives off water retention.

46. Malaysian laksa

100 g/4 oz rice vermicelli

600 ml/1 pint/2 cups chicken stock (broth)

1 handful fresh coriander leaves, chopped

1 shallot, chopped

1 scant handful shredded cooked chicken

1 handful prawns (shrimps), cooked and peeled*

1 tbsp coconut cream cut from a solid block

2 tbsp crunchy organic peanut butter

1 clove garlic, chopped

1 tsp Thai red curry paste (more if you like it hotter)

1 tbsp groundnut oil

Low-sodium salt

Garnish: fresh coriander leaves (cilantro)

* Defrost the prawns if frozen.

Heat the oil in a heavy-based saucepan, add the chopped shallot and garlic, and stir-fry for a few minutes until beginning to soften. Stir in the curry paste, followed by the stock, and bring to the boil. Turn down the heat, stir in the coconut cream and peanut butter and whisk to ensure they dissolve thoroughly. Add the chopped coriander leaves and cooked chicken, check the seasoning and add a little salt if necessary or some more curry paste. Be cautious with the salt, as the stock and/or peanut butter may already be salted.

Simmer gently for five minutes while you prepare the rice vermicelli according to the directions on the packet. When the vermicelli is ready, drain it thoroughly and place in a serving bowl. Stir the prawns into the soup and heat through for no more than 30 seconds, otherwise they may become tough. Ladle the soup over the vermicelli and serve garnished with fresh coriander leaves.

What it's good for

Like chicken and prawns, peanuts are a good source of protein and zinc. They are also rich in the amino acid arginine. The body needs arginine to make nitric oxide, which helps blood vessels to relax and so is beneficial for people with a tendency to high blood pressure. Farming practices that involve rotating peanut crops with cotton crops can lead to increased levels of pesticide in peanuts, so for health-conscious people an organic brand is recommended.

There is some interesting research which suggests that coriander leaves may be able to accelerate the excretion of toxic metals, such as lead, mercury and aluminium, from the body.

47. Mexican bean and lime soup with tofu

4 SERVINGS

450 g/1 lb/2 cups cooked pinto beans*

1.2 litres/2 pints/4 cups hot vegetable or chicken stock (broth)[†]

4 fresh tomatoes, skinned and chopped[§]

1 large onion, chopped

1 lime

225 g/8 oz tofu, cut into 1 cm/½ inch dice[v]

2 green hot chilli peppers, cut into long, thin strips

4 cloves garlic, crushed

2 tbsp fresh coriander leaf (cilantro), chopped

2 tbsp extra-virgin olive oil

1 tbsp tamari sauce[††]

1 tsp black mustard seeds

1 tsp ground paprika

Low-sodium salt

Garnish: fresh coriander leaves

* See page 271 or use canned beans that have been rinsed and drained.

[†] During the four-day detox, avoid using salted stock and try not to add salt to this soup.

[§] To skin tomatoes, leave them in a bowl of boiling water for 60 seconds, then drain and rinse with cold water. Use a sharp knife to remove the peel, which should come off easily.

[v] Use a chewy brand such as Cauldron.

[††] A high-quality, gluten-free soy sauce available from health-food stores and macrobiotic suppliers.

Scrub the lime under hot water to remove any wax. Finely grate 1 tsp of zest off the lime and reserve to one side. Now cut the ends off the lime, stand the lime on one end and use a sharp knife with a downward movement to cut off the peel all the way around. Now cut in between the membranes and remove the lime segments. Cut these in half and reserve to one side.

Roughly mash the beans, using a fork or a potato masher. Heat the olive oil over a medium heat in a large, shallow saucepan, and add the mustard seeds. When they begin to pop, stir in the chopped onion, 3½ cloves of the crushed garlic, and the chilli pepper strips.

Stir-fry until they soften, then add the lime zest and the mashed beans, and stir-fry until the beans become soft and creamy. Now stir in about a cupful of the hot stock. When this has been incorporated, stir in the rest, followed by the chopped coriander. Bring to simmering point and simmer for 15 minutes, stirring occasionally. Finally stir in the tofu, paprika, chopped tomatoes, lime flesh, tamari sauce and the rest of the garlic. Taste the soup and add a little salt if necessary (you may not need any if you used a stock cube). Turn off the heat, cover the pan and leave to heat through for two minutes. Before serving, garnish the soup with fresh coriander leaves.

What it's good for

Here are just a few health benefits provided by this soup. Beans: rich in protein, B-vitamins and minerals. Tomatoes: rich in the anti-cancer carotene lycopene. Raw garlic: has blood sterilizing, antifungal and anti-cancer action. Onion: contains quercetin, which fights allergies and viruses and helps to prevent cancer. Lime: rich in vitamin C and flavonoids, which help to strengthen blood vessels. As a natural soy food with little processing, tofu has many health benefits, including significant cholesterol-lowering properties and as an aid to preventing breast and prostate cancers. The warmth of chillies aids the microcirculation and, according to Oriental medicine, also helps to burn off water retention.

48. Moroccan chickpea chorba

2 x 400 g/14 oz cans of chickpeas, rinsed and drained
OR 450 g/1 lb/2 generous cups home-cooked chickpeas
   (see page 271)
4 portions organic chicken, skinned
2 medium potatoes, peeled and diced
1 medium onion, grated
1 handful fresh parsley, chopped
4 tbsp olive oil
1 small can of tomato purée (paste)
1 tbsp lemon juice
2 tsp powdered dried ginger
1 tsp turmeric
Low-sodium salt
Boiling water
Garnish: fresh mint leaves and tomato slices

Make a paste with the olive oil, turmeric and ginger. Put the chicken portions in a saucepan large enough to hold them all in one layer. Pour over them just enough boiling water to cover, and place over a high heat. Bring back to the boil, stir in the olive oil paste and simmer gently with the lid on for one hour.

Remove the pan from the heat, take out the chicken pieces and put to one side. Now place the chickpeas, potatoes, onion, tomato purée, lemon juice and parsley in the saucepan, stir well and return to the heat. If necessary, top up with just enough boiling water to cover the ingredients. (Stir the ingredients to help them collapse as you add the water a little at a time.) Bring back to the boil and simmer for 40 minutes.

Meanwhile, remove the chicken flesh from the bones, cut into bite-sized chunks and discard the bones. Just before serving, fold the chicken meat into the other ingredients and warm through for a few minutes. Taste the soup and add a little salt if necessary. Serve in a wide, shallow dish, garnished with chopped fresh mint leaves and slices of fresh tomato.

What it's good for

Turmeric has numerous health benefits. It contains one of the most powerful known antioxidants, curcumin, which gives turmeric its deep-yellow colour. Turmeric has anti-arthritis and liver-protective properties. It assists liver drainage and repair, boosts glutathione, and has even been used to treat hepatitis.

Chickpeas are dense and filling yet rich in dietary fibre, which helps to slow down carbohydrate absorption.

In Oriental medicine, the warmth of dried ginger is considered to help boost metabolism and drive water retention out of the body. Ginger is also an excellent digestive aid.

49. Mung bean soup with garlic and ginger

2-3 SERVINGS

150 ml/5 fl oz/½ cup dried mung beans (measured in a
   measuring jug)
2 cups boiling water
1 cm/½ inch knob of fresh ginger, peeled and finely shredded
2 cloves garlic, crushed
2 tbsp olive oil
1 small chilli pepper, deseeded and finely chopped
1 tbsp lemon juice
1 tbsp fresh coriander leaves (cilantro), chopped
1 tsp tahini*
Low-sodium salt

* Tahini is a paste made from sesame seeds and is available from health-food
stores or shops that sell Greek, Turkish and Middle Eastern foods.

Place the beans and water in a saucepan and bring to the boil over a
high heat. Turn down the heat, cover the pan and simmer gently for 45
minutes or until the beans are tender and beginning to get mushy.
Remove from the heat. Using the back of a spoon, mash and stir the
beans until the soup begins to thicken. Stir in the tahini and ensure it
dissolves.

While the beans are cooking, heat the olive oil in a small pan over a
medium heat and add the ginger, garlic and chopped chilli pepper. Stir-
fry until the garlic is soft but not brown. Remove from the heat.

When the beans are ready, stir the lemon juice, chopped coriander
and the fried garlic, ginger and chilli into the beans. Stir in a little more
boiling water until you get the consistency you prefer. Before serving,
taste the soup and add a little salt if necessary.

What it's good for

Mung beans are rich in B-vitamins, iron, zinc and soluble fibre. In Oriental medicine, it is believed that they have a cooling, soothing effect on a hot constitution. They are especially good if you are a person who tends to suffer from fevers and skin eruptions, and if you feel the heat easily.

The warmth of the ginger and chilli pepper in this recipe helps to balance the cooling quality of the beans. Sesame seeds are rich in calcium, magnesium, fibre and essential polyunsaturated oils.

50. Paraguayan zucchini soup with egg

1.2 litres/2 pints/4 cups vegetable or chicken stock (broth)

4 large courgettes (zucchini), coarsely grated

1 onion, finely chopped

2 tbsp brown rice

2 cloves garlic, chopped

1 egg

2 tbsp olive oil

Low-sodium salt and freshly ground black pepper

Heat the olive oil in a saucepan over a medium heat, add the onion and garlic, and stir-fry until beginning to soften. Stir in the rice, then pour in the stock and bring to the boil. Simmer over a low heat for 25 minutes, then stir in the grated courgettes, bring back to the boil and simmer for a further five minutes. Check the seasoning and add a little salt if necessary (you may not need any if you used a stock cube).

Crack the egg into a bowl, and whisk it. Pour the egg into the soup in a thin stream, while gently stirring the soup in a clockwise direction (anticlockwise if you are left-handed). Remove the pan from the heat, taste the soup and add a little salt if necessary. Serve seasoned with freshly ground black pepper.

Variation

Stir in a handful of shredded spinach with the courgettes.

What it's good for

Egg is a good source of protein and is rather underused in soup recipes. Egg yolk also provides nutrients such as zinc and a little vitamin A, D and E. Although egg yolks contain cholesterol, it is the cholesterol made within the body as a result of eating too little fibre and too much sugar and animal fat which mostly clogs arteries. In fact, the American Heart Association approves an intake of up to four eggs a week.

Brown rice is a good source of B-vitamins, and rice itself also provides protein. Courgettes are a good source of potassium and fibre.

51. Potato and walnut pesto soup with tofu

2 SERVINGS

3 medium potatoes

1 medium onion*

110 g/4 oz firm tofu, diced and mopped dry with kitchen paper†

1 handful fresh basil leaves

2 tbsp lime juice

1 tbsp walnuts

2 cloves garlic

4 tbsp olive oil

½ tsp sea salt

Boiling water

Garnish: sprouted seeds§ and a little grated carrot

* Don't use a red onion for this recipe as it will affect the colour.

† Use a chewy brand of tofu, such as Cauldron. Avoid silken tofu for this recipe.

§ See page 273 for how to prepare these. Sprouted seeds can also be purchased from some health-food stores.

Using a mortar and pestle, make a pesto by pounding the basil, garlic, salt and walnuts into a paste with 2 tbsp olive oil. Alternatively, you may find it easier to pound the salt, garlic and walnuts first, and then process them with the olive oil and basil leaves in a mini food processor. Scrape the pesto into a bowl, and add the lime juice and the diced tofu. Stir the tofu until it is well coated, adding a little more olive oil if necessary. Leave to marinate while you follow the rest of the recipe.

Peel the onion and cut it in half lengthwise. Then thinly slice it lengthwise. Peel the potatoes and cut into quarters lengthwise. Then cut into thin slices.

Sweat the onion in a large saucepan with 2 tbsp olive oil until beginning to soften, then add the potatoes and stir-fry for two minutes. Add just enough boiling water to cover the ingredients. Put a lid on the pan, bring it to the boil and simmer gently for 40 minutes, until the potatoes break up easily when stirred. Turn the heat down to its lowest setting and gently stir in the tofu and its marinade. Leave to steep and warm through for a minute before serving. Check the consistency – if the soup is too thick for your liking, stir in a little more hot water. Taste the soup and add a little more salt if necessary. Serve garnished with a little pile of sprouted seeds in the centre and some shreds of grated carrot.

What it's good for

The garlic in this recipe is nearly raw, giving it antibacterial and antifungal properties which help to combat imbalances in intestinal bacteria. Olive oil also has antifungal properties. Tofu is a good source of vegetarian protein. Being made from soy, it helps to combat high cholesterol and also female problems related to excessively high oestrogen levels.

52. Red lentil and chestnut soup

2–4 SERVINGS

150 ml/5 fl oz/½ cup red lentils (measured in a measuring jug)

600 ml/1 pint/2 cups boiling water

1 x 200 g/7 oz pack of vacuum-packed chestnuts*

1 medium red onion, chopped

2 tbsp olive oil

1 tbsp brown rice miso dissolved in 1 cup of boiling water

1 tbsp lemon juice

1 tbsp fresh parsley, chopped

½ tsp cumin seeds and ½ tsp fenugreek seeds, roughly crushed
    with a mortar and pestle

Low-sodium salt and freshly ground black pepper

* You could also use dried chestnuts. They will need prior soaking overnight followed by boiling until tender. Fresh chestnuts need to be boiled until tender and then peeled while still hot.

Fry the onions in the olive oil over a medium heat until beginning to soften. Add the cumin and fenugreek seeds and stir-fry for one minute. Put the water and lentils in a saucepan and bring to the boil, then stir in the onions. Bring to the boil and simmer gently for 35 minutes, stirring occasionally.

Stir the miso liquid into the pan. Squash the chestnuts gently with the heel of your hand to break them up a little, then add them to the pan. Simmer for five more minutes, then stir in the lemon juice and parsley. Taste the soup and add a little salt if necessary (miso already contains salt). Season with black pepper before serving.

What it's good for

The colour in red onions is a natural pigment known as anthocyanin, which is a good antioxidant. Chestnuts are low in oil and rich in carbo-hydrate – nutritionally quite similar to grains such as corn or rice. Deli-ciously sweet, they are a good source of potassium, magnesium and iron. Lentils are a good source of folic acid and iron. The lemon juice and the vitamin C in the fresh parsley will help you to absorb the iron. Fenugreek seeds are a natural lubricant for the large intestine and have a soothing effect on the digestive system in general.

53. Salmon and potato chunky chowder

225 g/8 oz fresh salmon, cut into bite-size chunks

4 medium potatoes, thinly sliced

3 large handfuls of finely shredded greens, e.g. savoy cabbage,
    greens, kale or other dark-green edible leaves*

Approx. 1 litre/1¾ pints/4 cups salmon fish stock (broth)†

1 large red onion, cut in half lengthwise, then thinly sliced
    lengthwise

4 tbsp olive oil

1 tsp powdered ginger

4 tbsp soy cream

Low-sodium salt

* To shred the leaves, remove any tough stalks, then roll them up and cut them crosswise into fine strips.

† Ask the fishmonger for salmon trimmings, such as heads and bones. Boil these in water for one hour, then strain.

Using a large, heavy-bottomed saucepan, fry the onion in the olive oil over a medium heat until tender and beginning to turn golden. Stir in the potatoes and press down. Put a lid on the pan to conserve the steam. Stir the contents of the pan every few minutes and press down again. When the potatoes are a little browned, stir in the greens. Replace the lid. Cook for a few more minutes, stirring from time to time, until the greens are wilted, then add the ginger and just enough fish stock to cover the contents of the pan. Stir, bring to a gentle simmer with the lid on and cook over a low heat for 25 minutes. Taste the soup and add a little salt if necessary.

Gently fold in the salmon chunks and cook for a further five minutes or until the fish flakes easily. Remove from the heat. Gently stir in the soy cream and serve the chowder in shallow bowls.

What it's good for

Salmon is classified as an 'oily' fish, which means that the flesh is a source of oils with many health benefits, especially for your circulation. Wild or organic salmon are best, since the nutritional value of fish does partly depend on what it is fed. Farmed salmon are fed with chemicals to make their flesh pink. (By contrast, organic farmed salmon have quite pale flesh.) The pink or red colour of wild salmon is due to the natural foods they eat in the wild.

54. Scallop and potato chowder

4 SERVINGS

250 g/generous ½ lb salad potatoes, unpeeled
2 cups mixed peas and sweetcorn kernels, either fresh or frozen*
8 fresh scallops (without shells)
4 shallots, peeled and cut into quarters lengthwise
1 cup soy or cow's milk
2 tbsp butter
1 slightly rounded tbsp rice flour or wheat flour
2 tbsp dairy or soy cream or crème fraîche
1 pinch dried tarragon
Low-sodium salt and freshly ground black pepper
Boiling water

* Frozen products containing diced carrots or other vegetables can also be used.

Boil the potatoes in their jackets until tender all the way through when tested with a knife (about 30–40 minutes, depending on size). Drain and plunge into a sink of cold water for a few minutes until they have cooled down enough to handle them. Drain the potatoes again, peel them and cut into bite-sized pieces. Reserve to one side.

While the potatoes are cooking, separate the red corals from the scallops. Cut off and discard any tough sinews. Slice the scallops across in half. Place the scallops and their corals in a small saucepan and add the milk. Bring to simmering point (watch the pan to ensure it does not boil over!) and simmer very gently with a lid on for two minutes until the scallops are cooked through. Remove from the heat. Using a slotted spoon, remove the scallops and place them in a bowl. Reserve the cooking liquid. Roughly chop the corals, replace them in the milk, and whizz with a hand blender until smooth.

Meanwhile, melt a tablespoon of butter in a saucepan, add the shallots plus two tablespoons of water, cover the pan and soften the shallots over a low to medium heat for five minutes. Do not allow them to brown. If necessary, add a little more water. When the shallots are tender, remove the lid and turn up the heat to evaporate the remains of the water. Sprinkle the flour over the shallots and keep stirring until it is absorbed. Then pour a cup of hot water into the pan, and continue to stir until the mixture thickens. Now add the liquidized corals and their milk, and stir in the peas, sweetcorn and tarragon. Bring the pan to a gentle simmer, cover it and simmer very gently for five minutes, stirring occasionally. Taste the soup and add a little salt if necessary.

Now stir in the cooked potatoes, scallop meat and cream, and gently heat through but do not allow to boil. Season with freshly ground black pepper before serving.

What it's good for

This gorgeous soup is very rich, and you probably will not be able to eat large portions of it. Scallops are seafood and therefore rich in the minerals of the sea: iodine, zinc, selenium and many other nutrients that can be sadly lacking in terrestrial foods. If you are on a wheat- and dairy-free diet such as the Waterfall Diet, simply use rice flour, soy milk and soy cream – you really won't notice the difference.

55. Seafood bisque cooked French-style

4 SERVINGS

450 g/1 lb cooked shellfish (with their shells)*

1.2 litres/2 pints/4 cups hot water

1 large potato, diced

1 onion, diced

1 large carrot, diced

1 stick of celery, chopped

4 cloves garlic, chopped

1 rounded tbsp rice or wheat flour

4 tbsp dairy or soy cream

4 tbsp butter

2 tbsp brandy

1 tbsp tomato purée (paste)

1 fresh bay leaf

1 sprig of thyme

½ tsp paprika

Sea salt and freshly ground black pepper

SPECIAL EQUIPMENT

A stainless steel pan is best when frying the shells, as their sharp
edges could damage non-stick coatings.

You will also need a very fine-mesh sieve.

* Crayfish, crab and lobster work well for this. A combination of dressed crab (the
fishmonger has scooped out all the flesh for you) and a few large prawns is quick
and easy.

Remove the shellfish meat from the shells and reserve to one side. Crush or cut up the shells into smallish pieces. (Use a hammer and a heavy-duty chopping block to break up tough shells such as crab and lobster.)

Melt 2 tbsp butter in a large, shallow saucepan over a medium heat, and add the shell pieces followed by the brandy. Stir-fry for two minutes, then stir in the hot water. Add the thyme and bay leaf and bring the pan to the boil. Cover and leave to simmer for 45 minutes.

Strain the contents of the saucepan through a very fine-mesh sieve into a measuring jug. To replace any water lost as steam, top up the jug with hot water to the original level.

Clean the saucepan, wipe it dry, then replace it over a medium heat and add the remaining 2 tbsp of butter. Add the onion, carrot, celery and garlic, and stir-fry until beginning to soften. Sprinkle with the flour and stir well to incorporate, then pour about a cupful of the hot shell stock into the pan and keep stirring until the mixture begins to thicken. Add the rest of the stock, and continue to stir. Now add the diced potato, paprika and tomato purée. If you are using crabmeat, put the brown meat into the soup now (continue to reserve the white meat). Simmer gently for 30 minutes, then remove from the heat.

Using a hand blender, whizz the soup until smooth, then stir in the cream and add the reserved meat from the shellfish. Season the bisque with a little salt, then replace it over a low heat to warm through for a few minutes without boiling. Just before serving, season with freshly ground black pepper.

What it's good for

Shellfish is an excellent source of minerals such as zinc and selenium which, in many parts of the world, are running low in plant foods. The shells are a very rich source of bone-building minerals such as calcium.

56. Soupe à la courgette (courgette soup, French-style)

2–4 SERVINGS

6 large courgettes (zucchini), diced
600 ml/1 pint/2 cups vegetable stock (broth)
2 cloves garlic, left whole
2 tbsp cream cheese or fromage frais
2 tbsp olive oil
Low-sodium salt and freshly ground black pepper

Using a wok or large frying pan, stir-fry the courgettes and garlic in the olive oil over a medium to high heat for about 10 minutes. They will begin to release water and soften. Transfer the contents of the pan to a saucepan and stir in the stock. Bring to simmering point, simmer for 10 minutes, then stir in the cream cheese or fromage frais. Use a hand blender to whizz until smooth. Taste the soup and add a little salt if necessary (you may not need any if you used a stock cube). Season with freshly ground black pepper before serving.

Soupe à la courgette is a traditional French soup, and ideal for using up a glut of courgettes in the summer. The technique is also suitable for other vegetables which become very soft when cooked, such as pumpkin, squash and sweet potato. You could also try it with celeriac.

What it's good for

From start to finish, this soup takes only about 30 minutes to make, but is loaded with vegetable goodness. Courgettes are a good source of potassium. Fromage frais is an excellent source of calcium.

57. Soupe de poisson (French fish soup)

1 kg/2½ lb fish fillets*

8–12 (depending on size) precooked shrimps (prawns) in their
  shells

1.2 litres/2 pints/4 cups fish stock (broth)†

Half a cup of white wine

1 bulb of fennel (with fronds), cut lengthwise into 8 wedges

2 sticks of celery, cut into 1 cm/½ inch segments

1 sweet red (bell) pepper, cut lengthwise into strips

2 tomatoes, skinned and cut into quarters§

1 medium onion (not red onion), cut in half lengthwise then sliced
  lengthwise

4 cloves garlic, chopped

1 small green chilli (seeds removed), finely chopped

4 tbsp olive oil

1 strip of orange rind, shredded

1 tbsp Pernod

1 tsp tomato purée (paste)

1 fresh bay leaf

1 sprig fresh thyme

Sea salt and freshly ground black pepper

* Use a mixture of different varieties and textures: cod or haddock, monkfish, red
snapper, sea bass or grey mullet.

† Make fish stock by keeping the trimmings left from filleting the fish. Boil these in
water for 30 minutes with a sachet of bouquet garni herbs, then strain.

§ To skin tomatoes, leave them in a bowl of boiling water for 60 seconds, then drain
and rinse with cold water. Use a sharp knife to remove the peel, which should come
off easily.

Chop and reserve the fronds from the fennel. Heat the olive oil in a large saucepan over a medium heat and add the fennel pieces, onion, celery, red pepper, garlic, orange rind and chilli. Stir together, turn the heat down, then place a lid on the pan and cook over a low heat for five minutes. Stir in the stock, white wine, Pernod and tomato purée, followed by the tomatoes, bay leaf and thyme. Bring to simmering point then simmer gently for 30 minutes.

Meanwhile, cut the fish fillets into equal bite-sized pieces measuring about 2.5 cm/1 inch square, so that they will all finish cooking at the same time. Stir the chopped fennel fronds into the soup. Add the cooked whole prawns to the pan, followed by the fish pieces. Replace the lid and poach for two minutes, then check that the fish is cooked through (it should be opaque and flake easily). Taste the soup and add a little salt if necessary. Season with freshly ground black pepper before serving.

What it's good for

The health benefits of fish are becoming more and more apparent as scientific research progresses. Partly due to its healthy oils (and lack of saturated fat), and partly to its mineral content (zinc, iodine and selenium in particular), fish is a genuine power food. It is especially beneficial for individuals with heart, artery or cholesterol problems.

58. Spinach and French lentil soup

1.2 litres/2 pints/4 cups water

150 g/5 oz/generous ½ cup Puy lentils* (or brown lentils if you
cannot get them)

225 g/8 oz/4 cups fresh spinach

1 large red onion, cut in half lengthwise then thinly sliced
lengthwise

4 tbsp olive oil

2 tbsp brown rice miso

1 tbsp tomato purée (paste)

1 tbsp fresh lemon juice

Low-sodium salt and freshly ground black pepper

* These are small green speckled lentils. They are best for this soup as they retain a
slightly chewy texture which contrasts well with the smoothness of the spinach.

Heat the olive oil in a large saucepan, then add the sliced onion and soften over a medium heat with the lid on, stirring occasionally. Add the water and lentils. Bring to the boil, then simmer gently for 30 minutes with the lid on the pan.

Meanwhile, wash the spinach in a bowl of cold water and drain in a colander. Twist off any tough, fibrous stalks from the spinach leaves, then take bundles of leaves and shred them coarsely with a knife. Turn the shredded spinach bundles round 90 degrees and shred crosswise so that the spinach ends up roughly chopped.

When the lentils are ready, stir in the miso and tomato purée (paste), and incorporate thoroughly, then stir in the spinach. Put the lid on and leave over a low heat for five minutes or until the spinach has wilted and softened.

Using a hand blender, briefly whizz the soup while still in the pan so that some of the lentils are still a little chewy, while the rest of the soup is smooth and thickened. Taste the soup and add a little salt if necessary. Stir in the lemon juice and freshly ground black pepper.

Variation

You can enhance the protein content of this soup by adding cubes of tofu. Don't use silken tofu for this recipe. Use a brand with a chewy texture, such as Cauldron.

What it's good for

Spinach and lentils are good sources of the important B-vitamin folic acid. Of all the vitamins, folic acid is most quickly lost when food is processed and stored. Folic acid helps to keep down levels of homocysteine, a cholesterol-raiser which has been linked with heart disease, Alzheimer's and other circulatory problems. Spinach is also an excellent source of iron, but remember that iron from plant foods is not well absorbed unless the meal also contains vitamin C. The lemon juice in this recipe will help you absorb the iron, and you could also finish the meal with some fresh fruit.

59. Sweet potato and groundnut soup

4 SERVINGS

1.2 litres/2 pints/4 cups vegetable stock (broth)

4 tbsp smooth, organic peanut butter

1 large onion, finely chopped

2 large sweet potatoes (preferably with orange flesh), peeled and
cut into 1 cm/½ inch dice

2 tbsp tomato purée (paste)

2 tbsp groundnut (peanut) oil

2 tbsp fresh coriander leaves (cilantro), chopped

2 small red chilli peppers, chopped

Low-sodium salt

Garnish: fresh coriander leaves

Heat the oil in a heavy-based saucepan, and stir-fry the onion and chillies until beginning to soften. Pour in the stock, add the sweet potatoes and tomato purée and stir well. Bring to the boil, cover the pan and simmer for 25 minutes. Add the chopped coriander and continue to simmer for another five minutes. Strain through a colander or sieve into a temporary container. Reserve the solids and pour the liquid back into the saucepan.

Now stir the peanut butter into the liquid and whisk (preferably using a balloon whisk) until it has all dissolved and has thickened the soup. Season with a little salt if necessary (the peanut butter and/or stock will probably contain some already). Pour the other ingredients back into the pan and gently stir to incorporate. Taste the soup and add a little salt if necessary. Heat through for a couple of minutes without allowing to boil. Serve garnished with fresh coriander leaves.

What it's good for

Organic peanut butter is used in this recipe because ordinary peanut crops are often rotated with cotton on the same soil. (Cotton tends to be treated with more toxic chemicals than are allowed for food.) Peanuts (also known as groundnuts) are a rich source of protein and monounsaturated oils. They also provide zinc and copper, and are a very good source of the amino acid arginine. The body needs arginine to make nitric oxide, which helps blood vessels to relax and so is beneficial for people with a tendency to high blood pressure.

The orange colour of sweet potatoes is due to their antioxidant carotenes.

60. Thai shrimp noodle soup

110 g/4 oz/scant 1 cup peeled shrimps*

100 g/4 oz rice vermicelli

600 ml/1 pint/2 cups hot water or shellfish stock (broth)†

6 cm/3 inch piece of white mooli radish (daikon), peeled and cut
    into matchsticks

1 small carrot, cut into matchsticks

1 cup fresh or frozen peas

1 medium onion, grated

1 small Thai chilli pepper, deseeded and finely chopped

2.5 cm/1 inch piece of fresh ginger, peeled and grated

2 cloves garlic, crushed or finely grated

1 handfuls fresh coriander leaves (cilantro), roughly chopped

1 tbsp red Thai curry paste

1 tbsp lime juice

Low-sodium salt

Boiling water

Garnish: coriander leaves

* In the UK, shrimps are known as prawns. For the best flavour, buy whole cooked
shrimps and peel them yourself. You can then use the shells to make the stock.
Otherwise you can use the frozen, ready-peeled variety. These should be defrosted
in a dish so that the defrost liquid is retained.

† To make stock, simmer the shells in water for 30 minutes, then strain.

Place the water or stock in a large saucepan. Add the carrot and radish sticks, grated onion, peas, coriander leaves, chilli and ginger, and bring to the boil. Turn down the heat and simmer for 10 minutes or until the carrot and radish pieces are tender.

Meanwhile, place the rice vermicelli in a bowl and cover with boiling water. Leave to soak until tender (2–5 minutes, depending on the fineness of the vermicelli), then drain. Rinse with cold water and drain again.

Stir the garlic, lime juice and curry paste into the soup, then the soaked vermicelli. Bring back to simmering point, then add the peeled shrimps (and their defrost juices, if applicable). If the shrimps were already cooked then turn off the heat and allow a couple of minutes for the shrimps to heat through before serving. If you used raw shrimps, continue simmering until they are just opaque, which means they are cooked. (Do not overcook shrimps or they will become tough.)

Taste the soup and add a little salt if necessary (shrimps are already a little salty). Garnish with fresh coriander leaves and serve immediately.

What it's good for

This soup contains several Yang tonics and digestive stimulants: shrimps, garlic, ginger, chillies, radish, onion. In Oriental medicine, Yang tonics are said to help drive water retention out of the body, aid weight-loss and boost vitality. This soup is also virtually fat-free, and seems to fill the body with a warm, light feeling. These spices also dissolve mucus and help to drive impurities from deep within your body; for instance, this soup often has an expectorant effect, helping to clean out your lungs.

61. Thai tom kha gai (chicken and vegetable) soup

4 SERVINGS

850 ml/1½ pints/3 cups Thai chicken stock (see below)

1 x 400 ml/14 fl oz can full-fat coconut milk*

225 g/8 oz organic raw chicken meat, cut into small bite-size pieces

A quarter of a medium-sized cabbage, finely shredded

15 cm/6 inch piece of white mooli radish (daikon), peeled and diced

8 small fresh Thai chillies

4 tbsp fresh lime juice

1 tbsp fish sauce

1 handful coriander leaves (cilantro), finely chopped

Low-sodium salt

TO MAKE THAI CHICKEN STOCK (BROTH)

1 cooked or raw carcass from an organic chicken

1 tsp powdered galangal

1 stalk fresh lemon grass, roughly crushed with a mortar and pestle

4 fresh kaffir lime leaves, rolled up and roughly crushed with a mortar and pestle

* Coconut milk is the juice squeezed from grated fresh coconut (the liquid that pours out when you crack open a coconut is called coconut water). The best brands of coconut milk often come from health-food or Asian shops, and consist of 55 per cent coconut extract with 45 per cent water. Stabilizers, thickeners or other additives are not necessary.

Place the chicken carcass in a pressure cooker and press down to compact it a little. Add the stock ingredients and cover the carcass with water. Over a high heat, bring to full pressure and cook for 25 minutes. Allow to cool without removing the lid, then strain while still warm.

If you don't have a pressure cooker, you can just simmer the ingredients for one hour in a covered saucepan, but this will not extract so much nutritional value.

Using a fork, prick the chillies firmly all the way along their length. This will release their flavour while keeping them whole so that you can avoid eating them if you wish (Thai chillies are extremely hot!). Place all the ingredients except the coriander leaves and salt in a saucepan and stir well together. Bring them to the boil, and simmer gently for 40 minutes or until the ingredients are tender and the chicken cooked through. Serve sprinkled with chopped coriander leaves. Taste the soup and add a little salt if necessary (fish sauce already contains some). If it is not spicy enough for your taste, add a few dashes of Tabasco sauce.

Variation

You can make a quick, easy version of this soup by using ordinary chicken stock made with a stock cube, and flavouring it with 2 tablespoons of Thai green curry paste. Replace the cabbage and radish with 4 cups of mixed chopped frozen vegetables, add the coconut milk, chicken pieces and lime juice, and simmer for 30–40 minutes. Not quite the real thing, but good if you're in a hurry!

What it's good for

Coconut contains oils that combat undesirable fungi in the intestines. With chillies and chicken, this is a warming soup, good for the circulation and the immune system and especially good for people lacking in energy. Boiling (and especially pressure-cooking) the carcass dissolves the cartilage and extracts glucosamine, which helps to combat arthritis. Radishes help to break down mucus and to balance the thyroid gland.

TIME-SAVING TIPS

Frozen rice, beans and lentils are a great standby. You can make a lot of really delicious fast recipes by combining these in different ways. Just add stock (broth), leftover cooked vegetables, fish or chicken, and you have a soup that's cheaper and far more nourishing than buying canned or packet products.

Frozen Brown Rice

You can buy brown rice from supermarkets and health-food stores. It is already used in some of the recipes in *The Big Healthy Soup Diet,* but you can save time by replacing uncooked rice with frozen cooked rice.

To prepare brown rice, wash well, then soak overnight in at least twice its volume of filtered water. When you are ready to cook the rice, rinse and drain it, place in a saucepan, add just enough water to barely cover the rice, bring it to the boil and then cover tightly and simmer on the lowest possible heat until tender (20–25 minutes). By now the water should all have been absorbed. If not, drain away any excess.

To freeze the rice, allow it to cool completely, then spread it out on an oiled baking tray and place in the freezer. Once frozen, the rice can be crumbled into grains and placed in freezer bags. (If you have difficulty, break it up as best you can, place in freezer bags and use a rolling pin or hammer to crush it while in the bag.)

Just add a handful of frozen brown rice to a pan of soup to give it extra body and substance.

Frozen Beans

It is always useful to keep a few cans of beans in your store cupboard, but buying dried beans and cooking them yourself can save you a lot of money. Once frozen and bagged, beans can be kept until you are ready to use a handful here and there to make a truly instant, easy soup.

If you are going to cook beans regularly, it really is worth investing in a pressure cooker. Some beans can take hours to cook if you don't have one, whereas a pressure cooker usually cuts the time down to 10 minutes at the most.

Dried beans should be soaked before cooking. Cover with four times their volume in boiling water and leave overnight.

The next day, throw away the soaking water, place the beans – well covered with fresh water – in a pressure cooker, bring to full steam, and leave on a low to medium heat for 3–10 minutes, depending on size and age. During this time, check that the steam pressure does not go down. If it does, turn the heat up a little.

After the cooking time, remove the pressure cooker from the heat and place it in a sink of cold water. You cannot open the pressure cooker until it has cooled down enough to reduce the steam pressure inside. Once you can open the pressure cooker, test a bean by eating it. It should be absolutely tender. If not, seal up the pressure cooker again and repeat the cooking process for a few minutes more.

Pressure-cooking breaks down the poisonous lectins found in raw beans. If you do not have a pressure cooker, boil them fast for at least 10 minutes before simmering or slow-cooking until tender.

To freeze beans, allow them to cool completely and follow the same method as for frozen brown rice (see page 271). Spoonfuls of split peas which are a little mushy can be frozen in the wells of tart or muffin baking tins before bagging.

Frozen Red Lentils – a Good Thickener

To cook red lentils, put them in a saucepan, add $2^1/_4$ times their volume of water, bring to the boil and simmer gently without a lid for 25 minutes. When the lentils are nearly cooked, they will thicken and you should keep stirring them to make sure they do not stick to the pan. When cooked, allow the lentils to cool. Now put the cooked lentils in ice cube trays and freeze them. Once frozen, you can put the cubes in freezer bags. Just pop a couple of frozen cubes into a pan of soup to thicken it. This tip is especially useful for individuals on low-carb diets.

GARNISHES

Sprouted Seeds

Use whole green or brown lentils, mung beans, aduki beans, radish seeds or alfalfa seeds. (You can often buy mixed seeds ready for sprouting from health-food stores.)

Place a tablespoon of seeds in a large jar, then cover the jar with a piece of nylon fabric from an old pair of tights and secure the fabric with an elastic band around the neck of the jar. Run some water into the jar, shake to thoroughly wet the seeds, then leave overnight. In the morning, pour the water away, straining it through the nylon cover. Rinse the seeds by pouring in water and immediately straining it out again morning and night, and in a few days you will have a luscious growth of curly green sprouts which can be added to soups or eaten as salad. Eat them when they are between 5 mm/$^1/_4$ inch and 2 cm/ 1 inch in length.

Other Garnishes

Many ideas are given in the recipes, but you could also use your own ideas. Try sliced spring onions (scallions), cheese cubes, flaked almonds, cashew nuts, sliced mushrooms (cooked or raw), thinly sliced tomatoes or pears, or celery leaves.

PART V

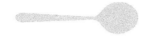

RESOURCES

Linda Lazarides' website

You can find extensive information about weight-loss and using food as medicine at Linda Lazarides' website: www.health-diets.net

The Waterfall Diet

Linda Lazarides' book, published by Piatkus Books (2003), is available from bookstores and online booksellers. *The Waterfall Diet* provides extensive information on water retention and its causes and treatment, and gives full instructions for the diet itself.

Psyllium husks

These can be ordered from health-food stores. There are many different brands, some left in their natural form and others powdered. The natural unpowdered ones are recommended for adding to soup as they are much cheaper and dissolve more easily. To thicken soup, whisk about one teaspoon of psyllium husks into each 600 ml/1 pint of liquid.

Organizations

These organizations can put you in touch with doctors and practitioners who use food as medicine.

United Kingdom

British Association for Nutritional Therapy
27 Old Gloucester St, London WC1N 3XX
Tel: 08706 061284
Email: theadministrator@bant.org.uk
www.bant.org.uk

British Society for Allergy, Environmental and Nutritional Medicine
PO Box 7, Knighton, Powys LD7 1WT
Information line: 0906 3020 010
www.bsaenm.org.

United States

American Academy of Environmental Medicine
7701 East Kellogg, Suite 625, Wichita, KS 67207, USA
Tel: (316) 684 5500
Email: administrator@aaem.com
www.aaem.com

Institute for Functional Medicine
4411 Pt. Fosdick Drive NW, Suite 305
PO Box 1697, Gig Harbor, WA 98335, USA
Tel: 800-228-0622
Email: client_services@fxmed.com
www.functionalmedicine.org

Australia

Australasian College of Nutritional and Environmental Medicine
13 Hilton St, Beaumaris, Vic 3193, Australia
Tel: +61 3 9589 6088
Email: mail@acnem.org
www.acnem.org

International

International Society for Orthomolecular Medicine
www.orthomed.org

INDEX

iodine 112–13, 116–17, 126, 155, 187, 219, 235, 255, 261
iron 9, 59, 69, 104
  cabbage soups 167
  cold soups 175
  hormones 112, 126
  one-pot meals 215, 229, 233, 237, 245, 251, 263
  special soups 141, 143, 155
  starters 189
irritable bowel syndrome 72
Italian tomato and parsley soup 190–1

Japanese buckwheat noodle soup 234–5
Jewish tradition 69
Johns Hopkins University 32
joints 53–4, 95–106
Journal of Acquired Immune Deficiency Syndrome 76
Journal of the American Medical Association 78, 91
Journal of Environmental Research 76
Journal of Nutritional and Environmental Medicine 106
Journal of Nutritional Medicine 64, 92, 103
juices 25, 49, 54, 68, 74, 88, 107, 114, 121
junk food 6–7, 109

Kaiser Permanente Center for Health Research 90
Keio University 105
kidneys 9, 13, 30, 45, 54, 67, 70, 119
King's College School of Medicine 64

laksa 238–9
The Lancet 126
leaky capillaries 85
lemons 251
  dal soup 236–7, 263
  soup 202–3
lentils 4, 8, 10, 37
  and chestnut soup 250–1
  circulation 86, 91
  frozen 273
  health 47
  hormones 109, 114, 122
  one-pot meals 237, 251, 263
  soup with roast peppers and apricots 214–15
ligaments 99
liquorice 49

liver 9, 13, 21, 25, 54, 57
  circulation 80, 87
  cold soups 175
  health 45
  hormones 111, 113–15, 118, 120, 122, 126
  immune system 68, 71
  one-pot meals 243
  special soups 155
Loma Lina University 47
London School of Hygiene and Tropical Medicine 47
Los Angeles Orthopedic Hospital 103
lupus 70, 72
lymphatic system 84–5

macrophages 69–70
magnesium 59, 64, 83–4, 92
  bones/joints 103–4
  cold soups 171
  fruit soups 139, 141, 143
  hormones 109, 120, 125, 127–8
  one-pot meals 245, 251
  special soups 155
  starters 209
Malaysian laksa 238–9
manganese 97, 104
margarine 5
marrowfat pea soup with sausage 230–1
meat 8, 10, 48, 56, 81, 91–2, 106, 114, 116
medicinal foods 54–5
Mediterranean diet 91, 93
Memorial University of Newfoundland 77
menopause 25, 97–8, 103–5, 108, 115, 117, 195
menstruation 85, 112, 115
mercury fillings 109
methionine 108–10, 115, 141, 153
Mexican bean and lime soup with tofu 240–1
Michigan State University 49
microcirculation 84–5, 93, 145, 203, 241
milk 10, 27, 43, 71, 96, 101, 116, 229
minerals 53–4, 66, 77, 83
  bones/joints 96, 99, 104
  hormones 107, 109, 112–13, 126
  one-pot meals 215, 219, 229, 231, 235, 241, 255, 257, 261
  special soups 155
  starters 187, 209

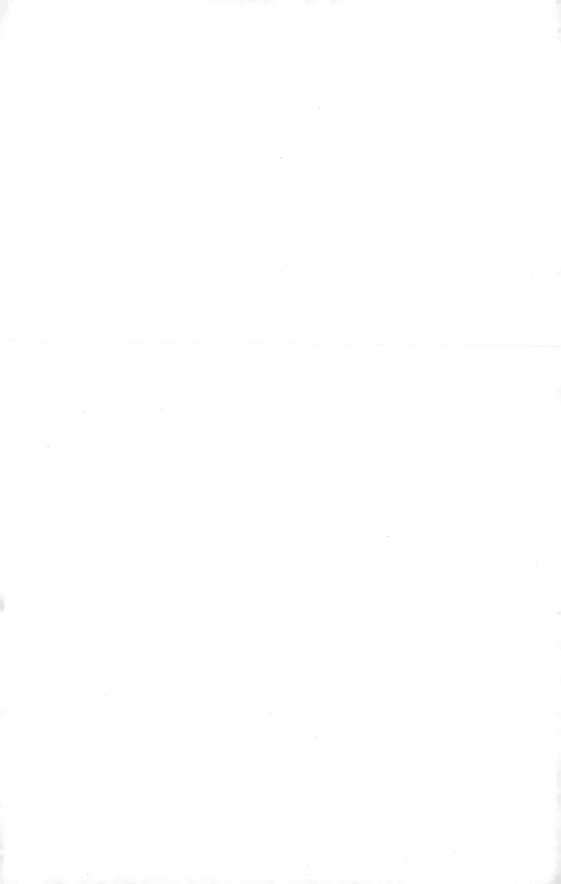

9 780007 207565